KRATOM IS MEDICINE

KRATOM IS MEDICINE

NATURAL RELIEF FOR ANXIETY, PAIN, FATIGUE, AND MORE

MICHELE ROSS, PHD

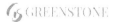

This book contains the opinions and ideas of its author and is intended to provide basic information about kratom. It is not intended to, nor does it, constitute medical, scientific, or other advice. If the reader needs personal medical, health, dietary, or other assistance or advice, the reader should consult a qualified healthcare professional. No claims, promises, or guarantees about the accuracy, completeness, or adequacy of the information contained in this book are made. Neither the author nor the publisher shall be liable or responsible for any injury, damage, or loss allegedly arising from any information or suggestions in this book.

Copyright © 2021 by Michele Ross, PhD. All rights reserved. Published in the United States by GreenStone Books.

www.greenstonebooks.com

The scanning, uploading, and distribution of this book without permission is a theft of the author's intellectual property. If you would like permission to use material from the book (other than for review purposes), please contact michele@kratomismedicine.com. Thank you for your support of the author's rights.

First Edition: February 2021

The author can reached for speaking engagements, media requests, and purchase of books at a bulk discount at drmicheleross.com/contact.

To all the patients, doctors, and industry professionals that have fought to keep kratom legal so that patients can access a safe and affordable option for pain management, thank you.

Pain is inevitable, suffering is optional.

- HARUKI MURAKAMI

CONTENTS

Introduction	1
How to Use This Book	8

PART 1
THE SCIENCE OF KRATOM

1. The Kratom Plant	13
2. The Opioid System	23
3. The Medicinal Benefits of Kratom Alkaloids	38
4. The Pharmacokinetics of Kratom Alkaloids	52

PART 2
KRATOM MEDICINE

5. The Safety Profile of Kratom	59
6. How To Use Kratom as Medicine	74
7. Medical Risks of Kratom Use	99
8. Potential Medical Applications of Kratom	111
Epilogue: The Secret To Success With Kratom	134
Acknowledgments	138
Appendix: Legal Risks of Kratom Use	140
Resources	145
Notes	147
Index	167
About the Author	171
Also by Dr. Michele Ross	173

INTRODUCTION

How many kratom users do you know? Probably none, because most don't proudly advertise their use. One scientist estimates there are at least 10 million kratom consumers in the Unites States alone, hiding in plain sight.[1] The highest number of searches on Google for kratom come from Portland, Oregon, and the average user is a middle class white woman.[2,3]

While plant medicines like CBD, cannabis, medicinal mushrooms, and even magic mushrooms are now being wildly embraced by patients and the media, kratom has been left behind as this taboo, dirty, opioid plant. CBD oil users are depicted in the media as health conscious moms who don't want to get high, cannabis users are split between sick medical marijuana patients and stoner bros looking to get as high as possible, and mushrooms users are depicted as enlightened patients looking to overcome trauma or addictions.

What comes to mind when you think of a kratom user? Do you even know what kratom is? If you do, you might think of a former heroin addict, using kratom to stay clean. You probably don't think of a mom with fibromyalgia, sipping on a cup of kratom tea for energy and pain relief.

AN UNEXPECTED CALLING

There's a lot of stigma still associated with kratom user due to the opioid epidemic, and new users are less likely to post on Facebook asking for help than say, someone looking for the best CBD oil brand. Most consumers trying out kratom for the first time are nervous. They're a bit scared of the fact that it's an opioid, and don't want to get addicted or die. They don't trust anything they read online, and they don't know anyone else who is a kratom user.

As a drug addiction neuroscientist, cannabis expert, and health coach, I was surprised to find the lack of solid guidance on where to buy kratom, how to use it, and the science behind it. As a patient with fibromyalgia, I just wanted to know how can I use this to stop my pain now, safely, with the least amount of side effects possible.

The kratom industry is today where the CBD industry was five years ago in terms of limited education and product availability, and where medical cannabis was ten years ago. I was one of the first cannabis educators and cannabis health coaches with a doctorate, and helped develop many of the original online articles, courses, and books on cannabis. Seeing the same gap in the kratom industry as a patient myself, I realized it was my turn to help educate kratom users.

I THOUGHT I WOULD NEVER TOUCH AN OPIOID

I grew up in a strict Catholic family in New Jersey and lived next door to a drug dealer who got lot of my classmates addicted to cocaine and pills. Since I was in middle school I wanted to be a doctor and end drug addiction. Fast forward to graduate school, where I was worked in a Molecular Psychiatry department studying the effects of "drugs of abuse" on the brain for the National Institute on Drug Abuse (NIDA).

While working on my PhD in Neuroscience, I helped rats give themselves intravenous drugs like cocaine or heroin in self-administration when they pressed the correct levers. Then I would collect their brains and study changes in cell number, cell function, or brain activity. Hundreds of brains later, I can tell you, taking heroin daily for hours is not good for the brain.

After graduating I moved from Dallas, Texas to Pasadena California to work at the California Institute of Technology as a postdoctoral research fellow. About three months into working at my new position, I got the call no one wants to hear. My little brother John had died in his sleep, from an alcohol and opioid overdose, at the age of 20. His death was so traumatizing, especially since as an addiction researcher I told him which drugs to avoid. I felt such guilt, like somehow I could have prevented it, even though that clearly wasn't the case.

Two months after his death I ended up picked to be the first scientist to star on reality television in 2009, on the show Big Brother 11. Afterwards, I quit my job at Caltech, got divorced, and navigated building a new career and life in Hollywood. I was surrounded by people struggling with anxiety, depression, and substance abuse. While I dabbled occasionally with some recreational drugs, I vowed never to touch an opioid pill or a line of heroin, not even once, no matter what celebrity I was hanging out with. My brother's death was always present in my mind.

AN ADDICTION SCIENTIST STRUGGLING WITH OPIOIDS

In 2013 my health started to downward spiral, with sudden bouts of muscle weakness, tremors, fatigue, headaches, severe nausea. After numerous ER visits and no one being able to give me a diagnosis, the mysterious cause of medical problems emerged.

My Los Angeles apartment was discovered to be covered

in black mold and multiple earthquakes had released lead paint all over, causing her to have heavy metal poisoning. I became wheelchair-bound, and barely survived multiple pulmonary embolisms (lung blood clots) that should have killed her over Christmas. The hospital called me their "Christmas miracle."

I began a long recovery process, including being on an oxygen tank, using a walker, and detoxing from heavy metals and black mold. I was diagnosed in 2015 with several chronic illnesses, including fibromyalgia and ovarian cysts, and struggled with prescription medications like Lyrica or morphine that marginally worked but had horrible side effects like sleepiness, insane weight gain, and addiction.

At one point I realized I was dependent on my morphine and oxycodone pills, and was getting horrible withdrawal symptoms in the morning when I woke up or if I took too long between doses. The opioid pills didn't even help with the pain anymore, they just stopped the opioid withdrawal symptoms. After my doctor refused to increase my dosages, I decided to quit opioids cold turkey. It was the worst 10 days of my life.

CANNABIS HELPED BUT SOMETHING WAS MISSING

My doctors had told me to give up on going back to work as a scientist, and apply for disability. They wanted me to accept chronic illness and my new homebound life. I refused and sought out alternative treatments to help me build strength, reduce pain, boost energy, and increase my cognitive abilities.

Sadly, natural alternatives barely worked as well or had their own set of unwanted side effects that made it difficult balancing my disease with working full-time and traveling around the world. Sorry, no amount of vitamin D or Ashwagandha is going to cure fibromyalgia.

CBD oil helped reduce inflammation and pain slightly, but was really equivalent to a Tylenol at best but was much more expensive for the level of pain I was dealing with. Smoking cannabis always made me dizzy and sleepy, or worse, anxious and hyper-focused on my pain. Edibles worked for sleep, but were illegal for me to travel with in many states and countries.

DISCOVERING KRATOM

I was introduced to kratom by a stranger on social media, but was concerned about the safety especially since it was an odd green powder in a Ziploc "baggie" that I didn't really know anything about.

I was told to buy a capsule machine and put the powder in capsules to swallow, which was a messy process that took hours I didn't have, and half the capsules broke in the process. Other ways to use kratom include putting the powder in a tissue and swallowing it with a drink, aka the "toss and wash" method of consuming kratom.

What? That's disgusting!

Some people put their kratom in coffee while others put their in hot water and drank it as a tea. No matter how many times I tried, coffee and plain kratom was nasty and I couldn't force myself to drink it. Kratom tea was like drinking grass juice with pulp in it. Utterly disgusting.

When I was able to use kratom capsules or tolerate drinking kratom, I found it was the only thing that worked for my severe fibromyalgia flares. Depending on the kratom strain I used, I either floated off to a solid 8 hours of quality sleep, or got a burst of energy so I could clean the house pain-free or focus on writing deadline.

WHY I FOUNDED AURA THERAPEUTICS

After months of experimenting with different kratom strains and ingredients, I stumbled upon a mood-boosting tea blend that was both delicious and effective for improving my quality of life with chronic illness. That horrible kratom taste was not only masked, but this "entourage effect" of ingredients appeared to potentiate the healing benefits of kratom.

I couldn't keep this secret to myself. I was ready to share my cup of AURA tea with the world! I wanted to smash the stigma of kratom and make women more at ease buying and using it. No more buying baggies of kratom from sketchy looking websites run by muscle heads or used car salesmen.

AURA is the first Dr. formulated functional beverage with kratom. It's made with lab-tested kratom and the highest quality ingredients, so you can feel safe purchasing from us. This year, we all could use a way to better handle stress and improve our well-being. Many people find a cup of AURA to be a relaxing and safer alternative to alcohol.

YOUR KRATOM STORY

Maybe kratom tea will become a trusted friend in your pantry. Or maybe it will be something you suggest to your best friend who is always dying from period pain. My goal with this book is to decrease the fear around kratom and open up both patients and clinicians to the possibility of using kratom for pain management and other wellness reasons.

Whether you're a patient looking to try kratom for the first time, or a clinician trying to understand your kratom-using patients better, this book shouldn't be your last point of education around kratom. At the Institute of Plant-Assisted Therapy, we offer patients consultations on kratom for patients, certifications in kratom coaching for professionals, an association for kratom clinicians, and a kratom research panel so we can fill in the gaps in knowledge to make kratom safer for all patients. Resources for both patients and professionals are provided at the end of the book.

HOW TO USE THIS BOOK

As a chronic pain patient and scientist, I understand both the need for scientific evidence to convince physicians, nurses, legislators, and other professionals about why kratom should be medicine, as well as the patient's need to cut to the chase and help them use it to get out of pain already.

The first part of this book explains the science of kratom and how it works in the body, and get a bit technical. You can skip to part two, kratom medicine, if you're limited on time or don't want to get too deep into the terminology and function of the chemicals in kratom. I do strongly encourage you to read part one when you do have time, as a strong understanding of the science of kratom will make you a better patient, clinician, or advocate.

Diving in deeper into Part 1, Chapter 1 discusses the history of the kratom plant and the many classes of chemical compounds found in it. Chapter 2 explains how the opioid system works, what the difference is between plant-based, animal-based, and synthetic opioids are, as well as how an opioid deficiency can impact the body. Chapter 3 goes over the major alkaloids present in kratom and how the work in the body. Chapter 4 elaborates on how bioavailable different alkaloids in kratom are and how they are metabolized in the body.

In Part 2, Chapter 5 examines how safe kratom sold in the United States is and how to properly store kratom. Chapter 6 provides a beginner's guide to the different kratom delivery methods, how to dose kratom, and how to handle potential side effects. Chapter 7 outlines who kratom may not be right for and how long-term use may cause damage in some patients. Chapter 8 delivers an overview over the medical conditions and symptoms kratom could potentially be beneficial in treating and the alkaloids that could be developed into pharmaceuticals for that purpose.

The Appendix includes a list of countries, states, and cities that have banned kratom. Check the Appendix first to make sure your location allows you to use kratom without criminal penalties. The Resources section provides links to to professional and community support for kratom users, as well as hotlines for potential kratom abuse or overdose.

The goal of this book is to help you understand if kratom might be the right option for you or a loved one. Please consult with your physician or an experienced kratom clinician before using kratom.

PART 1

THE SCIENCE OF KRATOM

CHAPTER 1

THE KRATOM PLANT

You don't need to need to a doctor, scientist, or health guru to understand the many health benefits of adding kratom to your life. But in order to make an educated decision about whether kratom is right for you, I am going to need to walk you through some difficult sounding chemistry and neuroscience terms. That's because unlike pharmaceutical prescriptions, which only contain one or two active ingredients at the most, kratom contains hundreds of chemicals.

Your first question when it comes to kratom is probably how to say it. While some people say KRAY-tum, others say KRAT-um. Either one is acceptable. Tomayto, tomahto! It is also called ketum or krathom in other countries. If you thought cannabis words were hard to say (hello cannabidivarin), kratom words can an even a bigger mouthful! The nice part is if you have some education in cannabis medicine, there are a lot of similar concepts in kratom medicine.

Kratom, known by its scientific name *Mitragyna speciosa*, is a tropical evergreen tree that grows naturally in Southeast Asian countries including Indonesia, Malaysia, Thailand, Myanmar, and Papua New Guinea. It belongs to the

Rubiaceae family which includes over 13,500 plants including the coffee plant. Dried kratom leaf is ground into powder and consumed in many different ways, from teas to capsules to vape cartridges.

If you have ever been to a marijuana dispensary you might be familiar with the fact that there are 1000s of cannabis strains, each with their own smell, effects, and silly name. There are less than 100 strains of kratom, but similar to cannabis, they each have their own unique chemical properties and benefits. Kratom contains chemical compounds that have both stimulant and opioid effects, making this a unique plant medicine that has been used safely for hundreds if not thousands of years.

The kratom plant is a cousin to the coffee tree, but it's much more complex when it comes to its chemical makeup. In fact, kratom is much more similar in complexity to *Cannabis sativa*, which has over 500 chemical compounds including over 100 cannabinoids. Kratom contains hundreds of compounds including over 50 alkaloids, terpenoids, flavonoids, tannins, saponins, and phenols.

WHAT ARE ALKALOIDS?

Alkaloids are the active ingredients in kratom, responsible for the feelings of euphoria, energy, focus, and pain relief depending on the dose taken. Scientifically, the term alkaloid refers to organic compounds containing at least one nitrogen atom and are usually basic as opposed to acidic.

Plants, animals, bacteria, and fungi can all produce alkaloids, and most have pharmacological activities in the human body. Plant-based alkaloids include caffeine, cocaine, morphine, psilocybin, nicotine, and mitragynine, which is the most abundant alkaloid in kratom. Phytocannabinoids like THC and CBD are not alkaloids.

Molecular structure of mitragynine

There are at least 54 alkaloids in kratom, although many are at such low levels they are nearly undetectable.[1] The most abundant alkaloids in kratom are mitragynine, 7-hydroxymitragynine, payantheine, speciogynine, and speciociliatine, while some of the minor alkaloids include mitraphylline, corynoxeine, speciophylline, and corynantheidine. The medicinal benefits of the most abundant alkaloids are reviewed in detail in chapter 4.

HOW THE KRATOM PLANT MAKES ALKALOIDS

The concentration of different alkaloids in kratom leaves depend on several factors including where the kratom plant is grown, the age of the plant when harvested, the timing of harvest, and if the plant has experienced any stress. Many plants, including kratom, express more of their active ingredient in response to stress to prevent their leaves from being eaten.[2]

Mitragynine is produced in the kratom plant in a complicated multistep process that is time-consuming and expensive to replicate in a factory setting, making synthetic mitragynine unfeasible as a pharmaceutical.[3] One of the building blocks of mitragynine is tryptophan, an amino acid that in humans, is also a building block of melatonin and serotonin. Feeding kratom plants tryptophan and other building blocks of alkaloids can increase the amount of alkaloids produced in the plant.

There are two main groups of kratom alkaloids based on their chemical structure: indole alkaloids and oxindole alkaloids. Mitragynine, paynantheine, and speciogynine belong to a group of corynanthe alkaloids, which are a large class of indole alkaloids. Most of the minor alkaloids in kratom are oxindole alkaloids. All three of the corynanthe alkaloids as well as 7-hydroxymitragynine have been synthesized chemically, but it is unclear how the plant makes many of the other alkaloids.[4] Only 13 of the 54 kratom alkaloids are available commercially as of 2019, and the purity of some of them is questionable.[5]

It is clear that more research on kratom cultivation as well as kratom alkaloid synthesis is necessary so that commercial producers of kratom can increase potency of specific alkaloids in strains, or bioengineer yeast to synthesize kratom alkaloids at a large scale. Kratom cultivation and manufacturing is in its early stages, and not as sophisticated as hemp, cannabis, or other crops.

DOES KRATOM HAVE AN ENTOURAGE EFFECT TOO?

The Entourage Effect theory, first posed by Dr. Raphael Mechoulam and Dr. Shimon Ben-Shabat in 1998 and expanded on by Dr. Ethan Russo, suggests that compounds in the cannabis plant such as cannabinoids, terpenes, and flavonoids work synergistically to deliver more medicinal benefits together than the sum of each of the isolated compounds.[6,7]

It is believed many botanical medicines, including magic mushrooms and kratom, also have an entourage effect whereby their numerous components work better together than an isolated extract of any active ingredient. This means taking kratom powder may be more effective for some symptoms than taking an extract of mitragynine, for example.

WHAT ARE TERPENOIDS?

Terpenoids are the largest class of chemicals extracted from plants. The term terpenoid is often used interchangeably with the word terpene, but in fact, these are two different compounds.

Many people are familiar with terpenes, the chemicals that give cannabis and essential oils their smell, flavor, and health benefits. When the chemicals are in the live plant, they are terpenes. When they have been exposed to oxygen, which happens in the process of drying cannabis flower for consumption, these terpenes are oxidized into terpenoids.

In a similar fashion, kratom contains terpenes in the living plant and terpenoids in the dried leaf powder. While over 20,000 terpenes have been found in nature, only around 200 have been found in the cannabis plant. How many terpenes have been identified so far in the kratom plant? Only two: ursolic acid and oleanic acid.[8]

Ursolic Acid
Ursolic acid is a triterpene found in vegetables and fruit with anti-inflammatory, antioxidant, anticancer, antibacterial, antifungal, and blood sugar normalizing health benefits.[9] One thing that's important to know it's not absorbed very well by the body when eaten, so it's possible many of the health benefits that are seen in research studies in petri dishes or in animals given shots may not translate to humans.

Oleanic Acid
Oleanic acid is a triterpene found in many plants and foods including olive oil. It has liver protecting, antiviral, and

antitumor properties, but also can reduce male fertility at high doses.[10,11]

WHAT ARE SAPONINS?

Saponin is Latin for "in soap," referring to the bitter taste of these plant chemicals and their foamy nature when stirred in water. They belong to a class of compounds called glycosides, which are sugars attached to another organic molecule. In this case, two saponins found in kratom are sugars attached to terpenoids, and are further classified as quinovic acid glycosides. They are quinovic acid 3-O-β-D-quinovopyranoside and quinovic acid 3-O-β-D-glucopyranoside (also known as quinovin glycoside C).[12] Little is known about their function in the human body.

Daucosterol
Another saponin in kratom, daucosterol, also known as eleutheroside A or sitogluside, is the glycoside of beta-sitosterol, a plant steroid. Like other plant steroids, daucosterol has benefits for brain health, gut health, fighting cancer. It appears to kill liver, lung, and prostate cancer cells by inducing apoptosis.[13,14,15] Daucosterol also acts as a neuroprotectant and may be helpful for stroke treatment.[16] Finally, daucosterol reduced inflammation, oxidative stress, and expression of pro-inflammatory cytokines as well as symptoms of colitis in mice.[17]

Other glycosides
Other glycosides found in kratom include 1-O-feruloyl-β-D-glucopyranoside, benzyl-βD-glucopyranoside, 3-oxo-α-ionyl-O-β-D-glucopyranoside, roseoside, vogeloside, and epivogeloside.[18] Roseoside has antioxidant, antitumor, and insulin-increasing activity, suggesting that even these minor

compounds contribute to the entourage effect of kratom as a botanical medicine.[19,20]

WHAT ARE FLAVONOIDS?

Many of the flavonoids found in the cannabis plant have also been found in the kratom plant. Interestingly, many of them also stimulate the endocannabinoid system, contributing to kratom's broad effects on the body beyond the opioid system.

The flavonoids in kratom include quercetin and its glycosides quercitrin, rutin, isoquercitrin, kaempferol, hyperoside, and quercetin-3-galactoside-7-rhamnoside, apigenin and its glycosides, and epicatechin.

Quercetin

Quercetin is found in all tea leaves including kratom as well as foods like onions and apples. It is highly bioavailable when eaten, and the average person consumes 16 mg of quercetin a day in food.[21,22] Quercetin has strong antioxidant and anticancer effects, specifically against colon cancer.[23]

Kratom may boost levels of your natural endocannabinoid anandamide, the "bliss molecule" as part of its mood-boosting properties. Quercetin is a weak inhibitor of the enzyme that breaks down endocannabinoids, FAAH, and increases the amount of cannabinoid receptors in your body.[24,25] When combined with kaempeferol, another flavonoid found in kratom, it reduces both pain and inflammation.[26]

Kaempferol

Kaempferol is found in all tea leaves including kratom, as well as broccoli and apples. It is highly bioavailable when eaten, and the average person consumes 5 mg of kaempferol a day in food.[27] Similar to quercetin, kaempferol also boosts activity of your body's endocannabinoid system by inhibiting the FAAH enzyme that normally breaks down levels of your bliss molecule anandamide.

Kaempferol is more than just a mood lifter. It's also an antioxidant, antiviral, antibacterial, anti-inflammatory, reducing diabetes risk, and may boost effects of antibiotics. It is also powerful against many forms of cancer, including breast, ovarian, pancreatic, lung, gastric and leukemia cancers.[28,29,30,31,32]

Apigenin

Apigenin is found in kratom and chamomile tea, as well as red wine, beer, cannabis, and many fruits, vegetables, and spices. It is one of the most well-researched flavonoids because of its powerful ability to prevent and kill cancers, including breast, colon, gastric, liver, lung, pancreatic, and prostate cancer.[33] Apigenin has other health benefits such as lowering stress levels, fighting inflammation, killing microbes, reducing symptoms of depression, and even reducing wrinkles when applied as a skin cream.

Epicatechin

Epicatechin is a flavonoid found in kratom, green tea, apples, berries, wine, and chocolate. It has been extensively studied for its anti-inflammatory properties and abilities to enhance muscle growth, promote blood flow during exercise, and offset the adverse effects of a high-fat diet on the heart and brain.[34]

WHAT ARE PHENOLS?

Plant polyphenols are of vast medical interest because of their antioxidant powers. Phenols are defined as chemical compounds that have one or more hydroxyl groups bonded to an aromatic hydrocarbon group. Kratom contains four polyphenols.

Caffeic Acid

Caffeic acid is a common polyphenol that is also found in all plants but is found ad moderate levels in coffee, wine, apples, pears, and artichokes. It has anti-inflammatory, antioxidant, antiviral, and anticancer effects, and is used to fight fatigue and boost the immune system.[35]

Chlorogenic Acid

Chlorogenic acid is also found in coffee, eggplants, peaches, and prunes. It's a powerful antioxidant, anti-inflammatory, antiviral, antibacterial, and can slightly reduce stress levels and blood pressure.[36] Popular green coffee bean extract supplements marketed for weight loss contain chlorogenic acid, suggesting that the chlorogenic acid in kratom may also be beneficial for weight management.

1-O-feruloyl-β-D-glucopyranoside

This polyphenol is an antioxidant that has not been throughly researched.

Benzyl-β-D-glucopyranoside

This polyphenol is also an antioxidant and the only paper published on its potential health benefits suggests it may ease stress in menopausal rats.[37]

WHAT ARE TANNINS?

Tannins are polyphenols that are found in kratom, tea, coffee, chocolate, and wine. They add to the bitter taste of kratom, but are also antioxidants and anti-inflammatory.[38] Recents studies suggest tannins also are beneficial for the heart and may improve the gut disorder Inflammatory Bowel Disease (IBD).[39]

SUMMARY

Kratom, like cannabis, is a complex botanical medicine with hundreds of active ingredients including alkaloids, flavonoids, phenols, and terpenoids that contribute to its potential health benefits. The individual chemicals likely contribute to an entourage effect that makes the full-plant extract more powerful than the sum of its individual components.

A major difference between kratom and cannabis include that kratom contains opioid-like alkaloids while cannabis has phytocannabinoids that activate the endocannabinoid system. Kratom also contains few terpenes, while cannabis strains are literally defined by combinations of their terpene content.

We're just starting to learn about the potential of kratom chemical components, and how their composition may help define both industry standards on kratom strain names as well medical applications. The future is exciting!

CHAPTER 2

THE OPIOID SYSTEM

The word "opioid" has been turned into a bad word recently due to the "opioid epidemic." When people hear the word, they think about addiction, overdose, and death by opiate drugs. What they don't realize is that opioids are made inside our body, and in many of the foods we eat. They don't realize how important our opioid system is to our health, or that an imbalance in opioid system function underlies many symptoms of chronic illness. Consuming plant-based opioids like those in kratom may be a new path to restoring health as well as providing an alternative to deadly prescription opioids for pain management.

WHAT IS THE OPIOID SYSTEM?

The opioid system is the neurotransmitter system consisting of endorphins and four types of opioid receptors including mu, delta, kappa, and nociception receptors. The opioid system regulates pain, mood, stress, and addiction, and is present in the brain, immune system, gut, and peripheral nervous system.

WHO HAS AN OPIOID SYSTEM?

Opiate receptors developed over 450 million years ago. Opiate receptors are not found in invertebrate animals or plants but are found in most vertebrate animals, including humans, rats, mice, frogs, cows, chickens, and fish.[1] It's possible opioid receptors evolved to help animals survive pain as well inflammation in response to injury, disease, or hunting by predators.[2]

WHY DO WE HAVE AN OPIOID SYSTEM?

While endorphins, or endogenous opioids, are produced in the body in response to pain, vigorous physical exercise, and stress, they are also produced in response to rewarding activities like sex or eating. More and more physiological functions are being attributed to the opioid system in recent years, making this system as important as the endocannabinoid system in terms of broad function.

The opioid system regulates:

- Nociception, the perception of noxious stimuli that is usually painful
- Analgesia, commonly known as pain relief
- Breathing
- Gastrointestinal activity
- Response to stress
- Expression of emotions
- Endocrine system activity
- Immune system function
- Pleasure
- Addictive behavior

The opioid system is truly the regulator of pleasure and pain. It's clear now that imbalances of the opioid system can results in chronic pain, mood issues, and addictive behaviors. The opioid system should be embraced and dysfunction quickly diagnosed, rather than making patients with chronic pain and other health issues feel stigmatized.

A BRIEF HISTORY OF OPIOID USE

Opioids have been used by humans for thousands of years. Scholars believe ancient Sumarians from around 3500 BC, living in what is now known as Iraq, were the first to use opium[3]. It likely was used to feel high during religious ceremonies. In the eight century traders brought opium to China and India, and between the tenth and thirteenth century opium spread through all of Europe.

Opium tolerance and addiction was first described in books from the sixteenth century, but efforts to ban the sale and use of opium failed in the seventeenth century. The active ingredient in opium was discovered in 1806 by Friedrich Sertürner and name morphine, after Morpheus, the god of dreams.[4] Morphine was then developed as an a common painkiller, but because it was found to be as addictive as opium, alternative opioids were developed. Heroin was created as a more potent version of morphine, and was supposedly non-addictive. That clearly was not the case.

Opioid drugs are considered one of history's most important medicines. Opioids like morphine were one of the only pain relievers available in the 19th century and also worked to suppress diarrhea and coughing. It was only in the 21st century did overprescribing of potent synthetic opioids like oxycontin lead to an increase in opioid dependence, overdose, and death, a period we describe as the Opioid Epidemic.

HOW DOES THE OPIOID SYSTEM WORK?

The opioid system consists of endogenous opioids called endorphins, opioid receptors, and enzymes that make and break down endorphins. While endorphins are often described as neurotransmitters, they are not. Endorphins are neuromodulators like hormones that impact signaling of a group on neurons, while neurotransmitters are released from one neuron, or brain cell, to another.

When a pain or stress is experienced, the spinal cord sends messages to the hypothalamus of the brain to make or release endorphins. These endorphins bind to opioid receptors on postsynaptic neurons in the brain. This causes downstream pathways to be activated, causing things like pain relief, pleasure, focus, and more. Endorphins work to increase the amount of dopamine released as well as reduce the amount of Substance P, a pain hormone, released.

While we make our own endogenous opioids, we can also ingest them from foods like milk or kratom, drugs like heroin, or medications like oxycontin. Each opioid different in how strongly it binds to opioid receptors, whether it also binds to other classes of receptors in the body like serotonin receptors, and whether it activates downstream pathways that result in respiratory depression and death. This is why some opioids cause mild pleasure, like those in cheese, while others are better at pain relief, like those in kratom, and others are highly addictive and dangerous, like fentanyl.

HOW ARE ENDORPHINS MADE?

Endogenous opioids are neuropeptides that are made primarily within the pituitary gland and hypothalamus of the brain. There are over 20 endorphins, divided into four classes: alpha-endorphins, beta-endorphins, gamma-endorphins, and sigma-endorphins. Beta-endorphins are the ones most commonly known for their role in exercise. All endorphins bind to the mu opioid receptor to produce feelings of euphoria and reduce pain.

A single precursor protein called proopiomelanocortin (POMC) is responsible for production of all endorphins. It is also the precursor for the stress hormone adrenocorticotropin hormone (ACTH). Endorphins are cut up and processed from POMC, and packaged in large dense core vesicles inside neurons in the hypothalamus and pituitary glands under they need to be released. Upon the correct chemical signals, they are secreted from the glands and flood the brain with pain relieving endorphins.

To make things slightly more complicated, endorphins are also stored in immune cells, which can travel to parts of the body that are injured and inflamed to release them.[5]

ARE THERE OTHER TYPES OF ENDOGENOUS OPIOIDS?

To keep it simple in this book, I refer to the endogenous opioids as endorphins, the most abundant opioid class which bind to the mu opioid receptor (MOR) and are responsible for most of the pleasurable and pain-relieving effects of our opioid system. However, there are many types of endogenous opioids produced int he body. Endomorphins also bind to MOR. Enkephalins bind to the delta opioid receptor (DOR), dynorphins bind to the kappa opioid receptor (KOR), and nociceptin binds to the nociceptin opioid receptor (NOR).[6]

WHERE ARE OPIOID RECEPTORS LOCATED?

Opioid receptors are like locks sitting on the cell membrane, and neurotransmitters, peptides, or hormones are the key that unlocks a chain reaction inside a cell, leading to physiological processes. There are four types of opioid receptors, although only the first three are known to be important for typical opioid system function: mu, delta, kappa, and nociceptin opioid receptors.

Until recently it was thought that opioids only activate receptors on the surface of cells. This is true for endorphins, but morphine and synthetic opioids also activate receptors inside the cell in an organelle called the Golgi apparatus[7]. It has been theorized that this mechanism may be one reason that prescription opioids are much more addictive than natural opioids like endorphins. It is not clear whether mitragynine and other alkaloids in kratom also activate the Golgi apparatus or they act more like endorphins once inside cells.

While some brain regions may express multiple types of opioid receptors, it is rare to see the same neuron express more than one type outside of the spinal cord.[8] This means, for example, that there are neurons with MORs and neurons with DORs, but rarely neurons with both. Below is a summary of where the different classes of opioid receptors are located, what physiological processes they are involved in, and what the medical benefits of agonists at these receptors are.

Mu opioid receptors (MOR)

MORs are distributed widely throughout the brain, including the brain stem, an area that controls breathing. This is why most opioids can cause respiratory depression and death, although kratom alkaloids are unique in that they don't activate the beta-arresting pathway in those neurons and can't cause death by respiratory depression by themselves.

The highest amounts of MORs are found in the in the dorsal horn of the spinal cord and these brain regions: nucleus accumbens, thalamus, caudate putamen, neocortex, amygdala, interpeduncular complex, inferior and superior colliculi, periaqueductal gray, and raphe nucleus. MORs play a role in pain and pain relief, mood, hormones, breathing, temperature regulation, feeding, gut function, heart health, and immune system function.[9]

Delta opioid receptors (DOR)
The highest amount of DORs are found in the dorsal horn of the spinal cord and these brain regions: neocortex, caudate putamen, nucleus accumbens, and amygdala, thalamus, and hypothalamus.[10] DORs play a role in pain relief, but other roles, like mood, gut function, and heart health are less researched.[11] Opioids that target DORs may have pain relieving, antidepressant, and anti-anxiety effects.[12]

Kappa opioid receptors (KOR)
The highest amounts of KORs are found in the cerebral cortex, nucleus accumbens, claustrum, and hypothalamus.[13] They play a role in pain perception, feeding, production of urine, neuroendocrine function, and immune system function.[14] Opioids that stimulate KORs can reduce inflammation, pain, and itching.[15]

Nociceptin opioid receptors (NOR)
NORs are not to be confused with nociception receptors or nociceptors. NORs do not bind to opioids in kratom or other opioid drugs, and only bind to nociceptin. NORs are expressed throughout dorsal horn of the spinal cord and the brain, and are highest in the cortex, amygdala, hippocampus, ventral tegmental area, hypothalamus, substantial nigra, locus coeuleus, and brain stem. They play a role in pain, pain relief, reward, feeding, mood, memory, gut function, heart health, and kidney health. NORs have a role in drug reward but nociceptin is not rewarding or addictive itself.[16]

EVERYONE'S OPIOID SYSTEM IS DIFFERENT

Two people in same amount of pain can have a different response to the same dose of opioid treatment because of factors like gender, body weight, liver health, genetic variations of the opioid system, and even where they are taking the opioid.

Mutations impact function

Genetics play a huge role in how our opioid system works. Single nucleotide polymorphisms (SNPs) are small mutations in genes that can cause differences in how proteins functions. There are over 17 SNPs in the gene for mu opioid receptor, OPRM1. The most common SNP in OPRM1 is called the G118 genotype, which causes beta-endorphins to bind 3 times as tightly to the receptor compared to people that have the normal version of the gene.[17] Another SNP in OPRM1, rs10485058, makes methadone treatment for opioid dependence less effective.[18]

Other SNPs that are important are ones in genes that metabolize the alkaloids in kratom, like p450 liver enzymes CYP3A4, CYP2D6, and CYP2C9. Some people have SNPs that make them fast metabolizers of drugs, while others are slow metabolizers and may feel the euphoric or sleep inducing effects of kratom more strongly.

The genetics of your opioid system

While commercial DNA tests like 23andMe can provide raw data on some SNPs in genes (and usually not all of them), you will need to important that data into a program like Promethease that can sift through the data and tell you what the SNPs you have mean for disease risk and function of different neurotransmitter systems, including the opioid system. For help interpreting your results, take your reports to a genetic counselor or functional medicine practitioner.

Will your genes impact how your body responds to kratom? Yes. Do we know exactly how all the different SNPs impact that response yet? Not entirely. If you want to geek out over the science of the opioid system and how your genetics impacts your response to kratom and other opioids, you can use the tools mentioned above. Don't worry, if this is too technical for you, you can still use kratom safely without knowing any of this.

ENDORPHIN DEFICIENCY

Because the opioid system is a neurotransmitter system, having too much or too little of our natural opioids, endorphins, can be a problem for our health. Endorphin deficiency is real, similar to endocannabinoid deficiency, dopamine deficiency, and other neurotransmitter imbalances. Endorphin deficiency can manifest as physical or mental health issues. Signs of endorphin deficiency include pain, anxiety, depression, substance abuse, and sleep issues.

While endorphin deficiency can be due to SNPs in genes that make opioid receptors, endorphins, or enzymes that make or break down endorphins, there are other factors at play including hormones, other medications taken, diet, and stress. Because women's menstrual cycles alter hormone and neurotransmitter levels, including endorphin levels, they are more prone to endorphin deficiency than men.

A unique opioid antagonist has begin to uncover the many health conditions where endorphin deficiency may play a role. Low dose naltrexone (LDN) works to block opioid receptors and force the body to produce more endorphins and enkephalins. It is currently used as a treatment for several chronic pain disorders, including fibromyalgia and temporomandibular joint syndrome (TMJ) as well as autoimmune disorders and cancer. Potentially every disease that LDN works for may have an endorphin or enkephalin deficiency component.

Endorphin deficiency is linked to the following medical conditions:

- Fibromyalgia[19,20]
- Depression[21]
- Anxiety[22]
- PTSD[23]
- Borderline personality disorder[24,25]
- Headache[26]
- Addiction
- Alcoholism
- Chronic pain
- Crohn's disease[27]
- Insomnia
- Bipolar disorder
- Schizophrenia
- HIV/AIDS[28]
- Cancer[29]

WAYS TO BOOST THE OPIOID SYSTEM NATURALLY

It's important to take care of your opioid system, whether you're healthy or have a chronic illness. Regular kratom users run the risk of decreasing their endorphin production over time, similar to how heavy cannabis users stop producing endocannabinoids like anandamide. What's different about endorphin deficiency and endocannabinoid deficiency is that is takes many more days to replenish endorphin levels that is does endocannabinoids.

Remember to take regular kratom tolerance breaks, and to engage in healthy ways to boost your endorphin production:

- breathe deeply
- eat raw cacao also known as dark chocolate
- eat delicious food, especially food rich in dairy or sugar
- eat spicy food
- exercise, in a group setting if possible
- orgasm, whether with a partner or by yourself
- laugh at a funny movie or TV show
- meditate
- inhale essential oils
- get a massage
- play with your children
- get acupuncture

IS KRATOM AN OPIOID OR OPIATE?

The words opioids and opiates are often used interchangeably in the media, but they are not the same.

Opioids
Opioids are any alkaloids that bind to opioid receptors in the brain. Endogenous opioids, or endorphins, are made in the body. Natural opioids are traditionally derived from the opium poppy. Semi-synthetic opioids such as morphine, heroin, oxycodone, and hydrocodone are synthesized from naturally occurring opium products. Fully synthetic opioids such as fentanyl, tramadol, and methadone are made entirely in the lab and do not occur in nature.

Opiates
Opiates are alkaloid drugs derived from the opium poppy including heroin, morphine, and codeine. Opiate is often used

interchangeably with opioid, but they are different, as opioids includes both natural and synthetic opioids, and opiate refers only to natural opioid drugs derived from the opium poppy.

The classification of botanical chemicals is confusing
Kratom is not derived from the opium poppy, so are kratom alkaloids opioids? Yes. **Kratom contains opioids**, but it is not an opiate drug. It's clear the language around opioids needs to be updated, as there are actually many exogenous opioids that don't fall in the traditional definitions.

Phytocannabinoids, or cannabinoids found in plants, have been discovered in many plants besides cannabis. Anandamide, an endogenous cannabinoid, was even found in truffle mushrooms, a food eaten by pigs and humans. Since truffles are fungi, and not plants, calling the anandamide in truffles a food-derived cannabinoid rather than a phytocannabinoid or endocannabinoid might be a more appropriate classification.

In the same way, opioids have been found in other plants and food products. We call them food-derived opioids. While some food-derived opioids are in their active form when consumed, like mitragynine in kratom, other foods contain proteins that turn into opioids when digested. An example of this is casein in milk. Even kratom has an opioid called mitragynine that turns into a more potent opioid mitragynine pseudoindoxyl when digested, making it a powerful food-derived opioid.

A suggested reclassification of opioid terms
As we discover more plant-based opioids and destigmatize the conversation around opioids in general, we will need the general public to clearly understand what each opioid term means.

I propose the following:

- *Endogenous opioids* - endorphins and other opioids made in the human body
- *Food-derived opioids* - opioids found in plant and animal food products including those in kratom, milk, wheat, soy, spinach, rice, and egg.
- *Opiates* - opioid drugs derived from the opium poppy including opium, codeine, morphine, heroin.
- *Synthetic opioids* - opioid drugs not derived from the opium poppy including oxycodone, oxycontin, tramadol, and fentanyl.

WHAT IS A NARCOTIC?

The term narcotic is derived from the Greek word for "stupor." The Drug Enforcement Administration (DEA) defines narcotics as opiates or synthetic opioids. Narcotics are controlled substances in the United States and many other countries, meaning it can be illegal to possess these drugs without a prescription.

The severity of these criminal penalties is dependent on the level that the drug is schedule on. Schedule 1 is the most restrictive level, and Schedule 5 is the least restrictive for controlled substances.

CONTROLLED SUBSTANCE SCHEDULES

Schedule 1

Schedule 1 drugs have no currently accepted medical use and a high potential for abuse. **Heroin** is the only opioid on this schedule, which also contains marijuana (cannabis), MDMA (ecstasy), peyote, LSD (acid) and methaqualone (Quaaludes).

Schedule 2

Schedule 2 drugs have a high potential for abuse and are likely to lead to severe psychological or physical dependence. Opioids that are on this schedule include **fentanyl, morphine, hydrocodone, oxycodone** (OxyContin), **hydromorphone** (Dilaudid), and **meperidine** (Demerol).

Schedule 3

Schedule 3 drugs have low to moderate potential for physical and psychological dependance. Painkillers containing the opiate drug codeine are on this schedule, including **Tylenol-Codeine** (Tylenol #3).

Schedule 4

Schedule 4 drugs have a low potential for abuse and low risk of dependence. The synthetic opioid **tramadol** is on this schedule.

Schedule 5

Schedule 5 drugs have a low potential for abuse and no or low levels of opiates in each dose. Cough suppressants containing low levels of the opiate drug codeine including **Robitussin AC** are on this schedule.

IS KRATOM A NARCOTIC?

Kratom is not a narcotic, and is not a scheduled drug in the United States on the federal level. That means a doctor's prescription is not required to posses or use kratom, and it is not illegal to manufacture or sell kratom. One caveat is that some states and cities have placed kratom on their drug schedules on a state level, restricting sales to minors under 21 and even criminalizing use or sales to all adults.

SUMMARY

It's clear opioids have had a huge impact on medicine over the years, and only recently have been hugely stigmatized. Kratom contains food-derived opioids that are legal federally in the United States and should be legal in each city and state.

Kratom has the ability to heal health disorders marked by endorphin deficiency, which range from chronic pain to autoimmune disorders to cancer to mental health and will be detailed in Chapter 8. In the next chapter I'll review exactly how the different opioids in kratom work in the body and what their potential health benefits may be.

CHAPTER 3

THE MEDICINAL BENEFITS OF KRATOM ALKALOIDS

Millions of people in the United States have used kratom, yet research on the medical benefits of kratom has had little funding. This is because most of the research funded has looked at the harms of using kratom.

Federal agencies like the DEA and NIDA hoped researchers would find kratom to be addictive and deadly, and they could place kratom on the controlled substance schedule as a Schedule 1 drug next to heroin. The short story? They were wrong. Studies have now confirmed its relative safety.

It's time to move beyond the minimal harms of kratom and focus on the medicinal benefits. It's frustrating as a clinician to know that it's still unclear what specific milligrams of kratom should be used for what type of symptom. While extensive research is still needed to look at the kratom strains and dosing that are most effective for relieving symptoms of medical conditions, there has been research on how individual alkaloids in kratom work in the body and what medical benefits they may have.

You may be familiar with how individual cannabinoids in cannabis, like CBD, THC, CBN, and CBG, are sold as separate extracts. Kratom alkaloids are not sold as separate extracts yet to the general public for consumption yet. It is possible that in the future, personalized blends of kratom alkaloid extracts could provide immense medical benefit to people with specific health conditions.

This chapter summarizes what we now about each alkaloid found in kratom, including the history of its discovery and research in test tubes, mice, and humans. Please remember that many of the minor alkaloids are present in very low amounts in kratom and may not not have clinically significant effects in humans at standard doses. Dosing, methods of administration, and other important information about how to use kratom as medicine are discussed in Chapter 6.

BASIC CONCEPTS

It's important to understand the science of how kratom alkaloids work. The term kratom opioids is not used here because may kratom alkaloids may activate other receptors outside the opioid system. Kratom alkaloids can directly activate or block neurotransmitter receptors, they can activate or block enzymes that build neurotransmitters, and they can activate or block enzymes that break down neurotransmitters. Kratom does so much more than simply activate your mu opioid receptors. Let's dive in.

MITRAGYNINE

Mitragynine is the most abundant chemical in the kratom plant, making up about 66% of the plant's total alkaloids. It was first discovered in 1921 by Scottish chemist Ellen Field. Mitragynine's chemical structure was mapped in 1964, the same year that THC, the active ingredient in cannabis, was.[1]

In the 1960s there was interest by the company now known as GlaxoSmithKilne in developing mitragynine as a painkiller to replace the opiate drug morphine. After it was found to be less potent than morphine at relieving pain and more comparable to the opiate codeine, drug manufacturers believed it could be marketed as an alternative to codeine. However, drug development ceased after a study found mitragynine was toxic to dogs.

Research on how mitragynine works in the body was slow because initially there was not enough material extracted to study in the lab. Other kratom alkaloids were isolated but not studied for decades due to lack of interest from pharmaceutical companies.

While mitragynine can cause mild euphoria, or a high, similar to opiate drugs or THC in cannabis, this does not mean medical users are trying to get high. The goal of responsible kratom users is to relieve pain, anxiety, depression, or other symptoms and still be functional. Because of the many ways mitragynine acts in the body, many users believe they are more focused and productive while using kratom that when they are not. My personal experience with kratom for fibromyalgia pain, fatigue, and brain fog as well as the experiences of my patients support this.

Some patients have medical conditions like fibromyalgia that reduce their ability to make endorphins in response to stress or injury. In these patients, consuming mitragynine as the major opioid in kratom to restore endorphin deficiency is a more natural and safer option than prescription opioids.

Scientific Research on Mitragynine (MG)
The numerous ways mitragynine works in the body are summarized here:

- *Mu opioid receptor (MOR)* - MG does not bind well with MOR in humans, and is sometimes reported as a partial agonist or even as an antagonist, blocking its activity.[2,3] That's very different from

morphine and other opioids which act as agonists, activating MOR strongly.
- *Delta opioid receptor (DOR)* - very weak antagonist
- *Kappa opioid receptor (KOR)* - competitive antagonist
- *Adrenergic receptors* - agonist at $α_{2A}$, $α_{2B}$, and $α_{2C}$ receptors
- *Adenosine receptors* - binds to A_{2a} receptors
- *Serotonin receptors* - antagonist at 5-HT_{2A} receptors[4], binds to 5-HT_{2C}, and 5-HT_7 receptors
- *Dopamine receptors* - binds to D2 receptor[5]
- *COX-2 enzymes* - inhibits the enzyme that makes prostaglandins which are chemicals that cause pain, inflammation, and fever.[6] COX-2 enzymes are produced in many types of cancer cells, and inhibiting COX-2 suppresses cancer growth and kills the cells.[7]

Medical Uses of Mitragynine
The medicinal benefits of mitragynine include:

- Anti-anxiety
- Analgesia
- Anticancer
- Antidepressant
- Antidiarrheal
- Anti-inflammatory
- Levels blood sugar
- Reduces cough
- Reduces high blood pressure
- Limited research, unclear if other uses

PAYNANTHEINE

Paynantheine make up about 8-9% of the total alkaloids in kratom, making it the second most abundant alkaloid after mitragynine. Since only mitragynine and 7-hydroxymitragynine are listed on kratom labels in terms of potency, many people don't even know that paynantheine is in their kratom or what it is. It's also much less researched than the two other alkaloids, which is concerning due to its high quantity in kratom.

Molecular structure of paynantheine

Scientific Research on Paynantheine
The numerous ways paynantheine works in the body are summarized here:

- *Mu opioid receptor (MOR)* - competitive antagonist[8]
- *Delta opioid receptor (DOR)* - no binding in humans
- *Acetylcholine receptors* - antagonist
- *Other non-opioid receptors* - unclear due to limited research[9]

Medical Uses of Paynantheine

The medicinal benefits of paynantheine include:

- Muscle relaxant[10]
- Limited research, unclear if other uses

SPECIOGYNINE

Speciogynine is the third most abundant kratom alkaloid after mitragynine and paynatheine, making up about 7% of the total plant alkaloids. Speciogynine is a stereoisomer of mitragynine, meaning it has the same chemical make up but the atoms are arranged differently in space.

Molecular structure of speciogynine

Scientific Research on Speciogynine

The numerous ways speciogynine works in the body are summarized here:

- *Mu opioid receptor (MOR)* - competitive antagonist[11]
- *Acetylcholine receptor* - antagonist
- *Adrenergic receptors* - no binding
- *Serotonin receptors* - possibly binds $5HT_{2A}$

- *Other non-opioid receptors* - unclear due to limited research

Medical Uses of Speciogynine

The medicinal benefits of speciogynine include:

- Muscle relaxant
- Limited research, unclear if other uses

7-HYDROXYMITRAGYNINE (7-OH)

7-hydroxymitragyine is the most potent alkaloid in the kratom plant but makes up only 2% of the plant alkaloids, landing at fourth place after mitragynine, paynantheine, and speciogynine. Although there is less of it in kratom than mitragynine, it is though to be the primary chemical responsible for the pain relieving and euphoric effects of kratom.

Molecular structure of 7-hydroxymitragynine

Scientific Research on 7-OH

The numerous ways 7-OH works in the body are summarized here:

- *Mu opioid receptor (MOR)* - 7-OH binds very well to

MOR but as a partial agonist, can block the receptors in the presence of stronger opioids like heroin. 7-OH binds to MOR nine times more strongly than MG.[12]
- *Delta opioid receptor (DOR)* - weak antagonist[13]
- *Kappa opioid receptor (KOR)* - competitive antagonist
- *Adrenergic receptors* - possible agonist at $α_{2A}$, $α_{2B}$, and $α_{2C}$ receptors
- *Other non-opioid receptors* - unclear due to limited research

Medical Uses of 7-OH

The medicinal benefits of 7-OH include:

- Analgesic - 7-OH is 13x more potent than morphine and 46x more potent than mitragynine.
- Limited research, unclear if other uses

SPECIOCILIATINE

Speciociliatine is the fifth most abundant alkaloid in some kratom strains, but others may have Cornyoxine B as as more abundant. Speciociliatine is a stereoisomer of mitragynine, having the same same chemical makeup but slightly different structure.

Molecular structure of speciociliatine

Scientific Research on Speciocilliatine

The numerous ways speciocilliatine works in the body are summarized here:

- *Mu opioid receptor (MOR)* - competitive antagonist[14]
- *Serotonin receptors* - possibly binds 5HT2A
- *Adrenergic receptors* - possible agonist at $α_{2A}$, $α_{2B,}$ and $α_{2C}$ receptors
- *Other non-opioid receptors* - unclear due to limited research

Medical Uses of Speciocilliatine

The medicinal benefits of speciocilliatine include:

- Analgesic
- Muscle relaxant
- Limited research, unclear if other uses

MITRAPHYLLINE

Mitraphylline is an alkaloid not normally abundant in kratom grown in its natural environment in Thailand and other Asian countries. However, kratom that was grown for research in the United States at the University of Mississippi was found to more mitraphylline than mitragynine content.[15] It's unclear how different temperatures, humidity, and cultivation techniques contributed to such a divergent expression of alkaloids.

Molecular structure of mitraphylline

Mitraphylline has been studied more extensively than some of the other minor alkaloids in kratom because it is present in high amounts in the herb *Uncaria tomentosa*, also known as Cat's Claw. Cat's Claw is used in Central and South America as indigenous medicine for over 2000 years.[16]

Scientific Research on Mitraphylline

The numerous ways mitraphylline works in the body are summarized here:

- *Mu opioid receptor (MOR)* - binds[17]
- *Delta opioid receptor (DOR)* - binds
- *Kappa opioid receptor (KOR)* - binds
- *Other non-opioid receptors* - unclear due to limited research

Medical Uses of Mitraphylline

The medicinal benefits of mitraphylline include:

- Alzheimer's disease[18]
- Anti-inflammatory
- Anti-cancer[19,20,21]
- Arthritis
- Asthma[22]
- Diuretic
- Heart disease
- Hypertensive (lowers blood pressure)
- Muscle relaxant
- Limited research, unclear if other uses

MITRAGYNINE PSEUDOINDOXYL

Mitragynine pseudoindoxyl is not an alkaloid found in the kratom plant, but it is a very potent and stable metabolite made when 7-OH is broken down in the bloodstream. This production of this alkaloid is comparable to how THC is broken down into the much more potent form 11-hydroxy-THC only when cannabis is consumed in edible form. I've left mitragynine pseudoindoxyl under the category of food-derived opioids because it is not made in the body, it has not been synthesized, and it can only be made after eating kratom.

Molecular structure of mitragynine pseudoindoxyl

CHEMICAL STRUCTURE OF KRATOM ALKALOIDS

There are many minor alkaloids in kratom that have not been quantified or studied extensively in terms of their activity at receptors or medicinal benefits.

There are two main groups of alkaloids: indole alkaloids and oxindole alkaloids. This differentiation is based on chemical structure, as indole alkaloids contain an indole and oxindole alkaloids contain an oxindole. We clearly know more about the indole alkaloids in kratom than the oxidnole alkaloids, even though oxindole alkaloids make up a significant amount of kratom alkaloids.

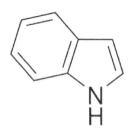

chemical structure of indole

Indole alkaloids in kratom

- Mitragynine
- 7-hydroxymitragynine
- Speciociliatine
- Speciogynine
- Mitraciliatine
- Paynantheine
- Isopaynantheine
- Isorhynchopylline
- Epiallo-Isopaynantheine
- Speciociliatine-N(4)-oxide
- Isopaynantheine-N(4)-oxide
- Epiallo-Isopaynantheine-N(4)-oxide

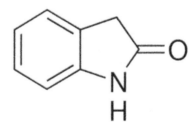

chemical structure of oxindole

Oxindole alkaloids in kratom

- Mitraphylline
- Speciofoline
- Isorotundifoleine
- Isospeciofoline
- Cornyoxine A
- Corynoxine B
- 3-epirhynchonphylline
- 3-epicorynonxine B
- Corynoxeine

SUMMARY

It is clear kratom is as complex of a plant as cannabis is, with its own entourage effect of numerous alkaloids that have activities both opioid receptors and non-opioid receptors. More research is needed on how abundant the minor alkaloids are in kratom as well as how they work in the body. The next chapter will review what we know about how the major kratom alkaloids are absorbed and metabolized in the body.

CHAPTER 4

THE PHARMACOKINETICS OF KRATOM ALKALOIDS

Pharmokinetics is the study of how drugs move the body. The journey of a drugs includes being absorbed by the body, reaching different organs to have intended effects, and being broken down and excreted out of the body. Because kratom is consumed in different ways, the delivery method can impact how much of the alkaloids are absorbed and metabolized.

Delivery methods include ingestion (capsules, tea, edibles, and "toss and wash" powder), sublingual tinctures, inhalation (smoking and vaping), and topical application (bath bombs, skin creams), all discussed in Chapter 6. The information provided here reviews the research on the pharmacokinetics of the most kratom alkaloids in the human body, including mitragynine, 7-hydroxymitragynine, payantheine, speciogynine, and speciociliatine.

MITRAGYNINE DISTRIBUTION AND METABOLISM

The primary method of consumption is drinking kratom tea or eating kratom capsules. When kratom is taken orally, the effects are usually felt within 10-30 minutes and last for 2-6 hours depending on the dose. Because mitragynine makes up 66% of the alkaloids found in kratom, it has been the most studied alkaloid in terms of bioavailability and metabolism. The pharmacokinetic results in humans are very different from rodent studies as well as a study in Beagle dogs, suggesting species differences in how kratom works.[1,2]

One study looked at 10 men who were regular users of kratom tea. It takes about 50 minutes for mitragynine to hit maximum levels in the bloodstream, but 85% of it is bound to plasma protein, making it unavailable to be bound to opioid receptors.[3]

After 23 hours, 50% of mitragynine is metabolized in the body, which is a much longer half life than most opioids.[4] It is broken down by p450 liver enzyme CYP3A4 into 7-OH, and by multiple p450 enzymes into 9-O-demethylmitragynine, 16-carboxymitragynine, 9-O-demethyl-16-carboxymitragynine.[5] While 7-OH is more potent as a metabolite than mitragynine, the other metabolites formed are weaker than mitragynine.[6] It's possible that patients are CYP3A4 fast metabolizers may convert more of the mitragynine into more potent 7-OH faster than slow metabolizers and therefore experience higher euphoria or sedative effects.

When kratom is ingested as powder or tea, only 0.14% of mitragynine consumed is found in urine. That means the majority of mitragynine is first-pass metabolized and turned into other chemicals, stored away from the bloodstream, or remains unchanged in the gut and is passed as feces. Similar to the lipophilic compounds in cannabis, THC and CBD, alkaloids in kratom are stored in fat tissue after 7 days of use.[7] 9-O-demethylmitragynine is the metabolite most abundant in urine.

One way that has been suggested to increase oral bioavailability of mitragynine is to turn it into a salt, similar to how cocaine in coca leaves is more bioavailable as cocaine hydrochloride. Chemically altering the structure of mitragynine makes it patentable and thus commercially viable for pharmaceutical development into a prescription drug. It is unclear what the bioavailability of delivery methods such as chewing kratom leaves, taking kratom tinctures sublingually, smoking or vaping kratom, using rectal suppositories, or applying transdermal patches. Smoking and vaping, sublingual administration, and rectal suppositories would avoid first pass metabolism in the liver, which would extend the time mitragynine is active in the system. In terms of topical application, mitragynine is lipophilic (fat soluble), and will be hard to penetrate the deep layers of skin and muscle tissue without additional ingredients.

7-HYDROXYMITRAGYNINE DISTRIBUTION AND METABOLISM

While there is significantly less 7-hydroxymitragynine (7-OH) in kratom than mitragynine (1% versus 66% of alkaloids), 7-OH is much more bioavailable when eaten and crosses the blood-brain-barrier more easily.[8] While 7-OH is found naturally in kratom, it can also be produced as a stronger metabolite of mitragynine after first pass metabolism in the liver. 7-OH itself is highly resistant to metabolism, with over 90% remaining after 40 minutes.[9] In rats, 7-OH is present in the blood even 8 hours after oral consumption.[10]

7-OH can be then be further metabolized in the bloodstream into mitragynine pseudoindoxyl, which is even more potent than 7-OH, but the mechanism of how it does it is unknown.[11] Because of this, it's unclear whether there is genetic variation in how mitragynine pseudoindoxyl is metabolized and if some people are at greater risk for kratom reward and addiction.

PAYANTHEINE DISTRIBUTION AND METABOLISM

The oral bioavailability of payantheine in humans has not been published, so it is unclear how well it is absorbed and distributed throughout the body. This is unfortunate because payantheine is the second most abundant alkaloid in kratom. In rats given kratom tea or a kratom shot, payantheine was seen in the blood one hour after consumption but not eight hours later, suggesting it is quickly metabolized in the rats.[12]

Payantheine (PAY) and its metabolites have been identified in human urine. These include: 9-O-demethyl PAY, 16-carboxy PAY, 17-carboxy-16,17-dihydro PAY, 9-O-demethyl PAY glucuronide, 9-O-demethyl PAY sulfate, and 16-carboxy PAY glucuronide.[13]

SPECIOGYNINE DISTRIBUTION AND METABOLISM

The oral bioavailability of speciogynine, the third most abundant alkaloid in kratom, has not been published. It is unclear how well it is absorbed and distributed throughout the human body. In rats, speciogynine is quickly metabolized and present one hour, but not eight hours, after oral consumption.[14]

Speciogynine (SG) and its metabolites have been identified in human urine. These include: 9-O-DMSG, 16-carboxy SG, 9-O-demethyl-16-carboxy SG, 17-O-demethyl-16,17-dihydro SG, 9,17-O-bisdemethyl-16,17-dihydro SG, 17-carboxy-16,17-dihydro SG, and 9-O-demethyl-17-carboxy-16,17-dihydro SG.[15] It is not clear if any of these speciogynine metabolites have any activity at opioid receptors.

SPECIOCILIATINE DISTRIBUTION AND METABOLISM

A recent study in rats found oral bioavailability of speciociliatine to be 20.7%, which is considered low, and has not been studied in humans yet.[16] Speciociliatine is both absorbed better and metabolized slower than kratom alkaloids mitragynine and corynantheidine, suggesting this alkaloid may be responsible for longer-lasting effects of kratom.[17] In rats, speciociliatine is still present in the blood 8 hours after oral kratom consumption, along with minor kratom alkaloid corynantheidine.[18] Speciociliatine and its metabolites have been identified in human urine.[19]

SUMMARY

More research needs to be performed on the pharmacokinetics of different delivery methods of kratom, including sublingual, topical, and vaping. In addition, most of the research has been performed in all male studies, which is not ideal as research suggests many drugs are metabolized differently in women. Finally, there is little research on bioavailability and metabolism of many of the minor alkaloids in kratom, which are just as important to the medicinal effects of kratom as mitragynine.

PART 2

KRATOM MEDICINE

CHAPTER 5

THE SAFETY PROFILE OF KRATOM

Kratom can really be thought of as the CBD of opioids when it comes to it safety profile. The safety of kratom is determined by three things: how the product is made, the health of the consumer, and how the consumer uses it. Education on what makes a product safe, who kratom might not be right for, and how to properly use kratom is key to reducing adverse effects, overdose, and in rare cases of polydrug use, death.

WHAT'S IN YOUR KRATOM?

Kratom is a new industry with gaps in regulation, and making sure you buy third-party lab tested products is the only way you can ensure you have a safe and effective product. What is third-party lab testing? It means that a lab that is not owned or operated by the kratom company tested the sample, so you can be confident that they are not lying about the results.

Look at the cannabis industry, where there is still a thriving black market of cheap, untested cannabis products and a legal, lab-tested industry that is regulated and often much more expensive. While it might seem like a bargain to get cheaper weed or vape pens, people have literally gone to the hospital because of adulterants in counterfeit vape pens and illegal pesticides sprayed on black market cannabis.

This same price versus health debate happens with kratom. You may be able to get cheap kratom online direct from farms in Indonesia through Facebook, instagram, or suspect sites. Remember that these suppliers are likely not lab-tested, and they may even show you a fake COA. Be smart and go with a tested and trusted kratom brand so you're not exposed to lead and other dangerous contaminants that could put you in the hospital.

How to find a Certificate of Analysis for kratom

When you're on a website shopping for kratom, looking for links in the header or footer menu for "lab testing," "quality assurance," "Certificate of Analysis," or "COA." Clicking on these links should pull up a page that tells you which lab performed their lab testing, and ideally, a pdf or image of their lab testing results. The Certificate of Analysis, or COA, should include the following information for kratom products:

- Potency of mitragynine and 7-hydroxymitragynine
- Presence of heavy metals
- Presence of bacteria (e.coli and salmonella)
- Presence of fungi (mold and yeast)

THE IMPORTANCE OF THIRD-PARTY LAB TESTING

Quality control is everything when it comes to kratom. The safety and quality of any supplement or food product is impacted by the soil its grown in, pesticides used, chemicals used in processing, and other variables such as the amount of heat, light, and oxygen it is exposed to during storage, packaging, and transportation. Poor manufacturing practices can lead to active ingredients no longer being effective, or worse, contamination with bacteria, mold, or chemicals that can make you sick or even kill you.

Why might kratom companies don't report third-party lab testing? It can be pretty expensive. A complete panel testing alkaloid potency, microbes, adulterants, and heavy metals can cost a vendor anywhere from $300 to $400 per batch of product for a COA. But the real reason is that companies know their source fails heavy metal or microbe testing, and still sell their products anyways. And that is scary.

The kratom industry is starting to self-regulate to ensure safety of products, make third-party lab testing the standard, and weed out bad industry actors. The American Kratom Association provides an AKA Good Manufacturing Practices (GMP) Qualified Kratom Vendor accreditation for kratom vendors that meet their standards.[1]

THE KRATOM CONSUMER PROTECTION ACT

The Kratom Consumer Protection Act (KCPA) is state legislation that regulates the kratom industry, making it safer for consumers to buy products and putting penalties on kratom vendors that don't follow regulations. In states where the KCPA is not passed, consumers can potentially buy unlabeled, untested, or worse, mislabeled products containing adulterants.

The American Kratom Association has been lobbied for the KCPA to replace kratom bans. The exact language in the KCPA may differ from state to state, but it usually includes the following regulations:

- Sales or gifting of kratom to a minor under the age of 18 is prohibited.

- The amount of kratom alkaloids mitragynine and 7-OH-mitragynine need to be listed on the package.
- Ingredients on the label need to be listed in descending order of how much are in the package.
- The name and mailing address of the manufacturer or distributor need to be listed on the package.
- Any directions or warnings about kratom consumption should be listed on the product label.

States that have passed the Kratom Consumer Protection Act:

- Utah
- Georgia
- Arizona
- Nevada

TESTING FOR ALKALOID POTENCY

The most eight abundant alkaloids in kratom are mitragynine, paynantheine, speciogynine, 7-hydroxymitragynine, speciociliatine, isopaynantheine, corynoxine A and corynonxine B. You might be surprised that only one or two of them, mitragynine and 7-hydroxymitragynine are tested for potency in most cases.

Kratom alkaloids are hard to identify in standard tests
Kratom alkaloid testing is usually performed by a method called high-performance liquid chromotagraphy (HPLC), which is the same method used for reporting cannabinoid potency in hemp or cannabis products. The difficulty in using this method for kratom is that many of the alkaloids are stereoisomers. This means they have the same chemical

makeup but different chemical structures, which results in the test not being able to tell the difference between these individual alkaloids.

Some COAs will report mitragynine and 7-hydroxymitragynine potency levels because they are able to be differentiated via HPLC, but then lump potency of all the other alkaloids together as "other alkaloids." Research scientists are able to find out the potency of the eight alkaloids and others in the kratom plant using alternate methods such as gas chromatography (GC) and supercritical fluid chromatography (SFC), but these methods are slow, expensive, or use equipment that is not available at traditional third-party lab testing sites.[2]

How alkaloid potency is reported on kratom products

States that have passed the Kratom Consumer Protection Act require the potency of kratom alkaloids mitragynine and 7-OH-mitragynine to be listed directly on the kratom package. This means that you don't have to go online to search for a COA on their website. Some even provide a QR code on the label you can with phone to pull up the full COA easily.

Potency of alkaloids is usually listed as a percentage of the total product, rather than by milligrams per gram (mg/g) or milligrams per milliliter (mg/mL), which is how cannabinoid potency is presented in cannabis. This makes reading a kratom label or kratom COA much easier than one for CBD oil or cannabis products.

What is the normal range for mitragynine potency?

Always check that your kratom has between 1-2% mitragynine potency. Most reputable brands won't sell kratom products that have less than 1% mitragynine in them, as that means the plant wasn't healthy or the active ingredient has degraded, and you won't feel effects like relaxation, energy, or pain relief after using it. On the flip side, having more than 2% mitragynine is unnatural and suggests your kratom vendor unethically added in mitragynine extract to make it more powerful.

What is the normal range for 7-hydroxymitragynine potency?
Always check that your kratom has between 0-1% 7-hydroxymitragynine potency. It is normal for their to be less 7-hydroxymitragynine than mitragynine in the product, and if there is more, that means that something is wrong and the product is adulterated. Unscrupulous kratom vendors sometimes add extra 7-hydroxymitragynine extract to kratom powder to make it extra strong for users who are looking to get high, and in some states, this is a criminal act.

Using potency testing for comparison shopping
Just like how the cannabinoids in cannabis can change based on time of harvesting, temperature, plant stress, and other variables, kratom alkaloids can also differ in the same strain from batch to batch even with the same vendor. Comparing the kratom alkaloid potencies for strains between different kratom vendors may tell you which one is stronger or perhaps a better value for your money.

If you use a certain strain and start to feel it's not working as well any more, you may want to use a strain that has a higher potency of 7-hydroxymitragynine or mitragynine.

The future of alkaloid potency testing
As we learn more about the medical benefits of the other alkaloids abundant in kratom, including paynantheine,

speciogynine, speciociliatine, isopaynantheine, corynoxine A and corynonxine B, it's clear potency levels are going to be desirable. It's likely that the combinations of different levels of alkaloids is what differentiates kratom strains. For medical applications, it will be important for consumers to be able to pick out a strain, for example, that is rich in the minor alkaloid that is cancer fighting.

TESTING FOR TERPENOID POTENCY

You may be familiar with terpene testing for cannabis. Beside CBD and THC potency, the potency of the 3-5 most abundant terpenes are often listed on the label now. The reasons for listing cannabis terpenes is many: they provide the smell and flavor of cannabis, they provide unique medicinal benefits, and the combination of terpenes present often verifies that a cannabis strain is labeled properly.

Terpene testing is not common with kratom products or required by the Kratom Consumer Protection Act, and for good reason. There are only two terpenes found in the kratom plant and two terpenoids found in the dried kratom leaf powder. The terpene content does not appear to change the flavor or effects of kratom, and thus is not something you have to worry about on a COA when it comes to your kratom products.

TESTING FOR HEAVY METALS

It's well known that the cannabis plant is a bioaccumulator, or plant that absorbs minerals and nutrients from the soil. Kratom is not common described as a bioaccumulator, but that is likely because it is not grown in the United States or researched as well as the cannabis plant, not because it doesn't have that feature.

Bioaccumlators can pull heavy metal like nickel, mercury, arsenic, lead, and cadmium from the ground, and it ingested by those who eat or smoke the plant. Heavy metals are not safe for human consumptions, and long-term exposure can cause nervous system damage, liver damage, headaches, high blood pressure, and even certain types of cancers.[3]

While hemp and cannabis regulations requiring heavy metal testing in most states has reduced the amount of products on the market with detectable heavy metal levels, this is still very much an issue with kratom products. The most common method of testing for heavy metals is mass spectroscopy (MS). The FDA tested 30 kratom products sold in the United States for heavy metals in 2019 and found almost all of them exceeded acceptable nickel and lead levels for daily oral consumption.[4] A third-party lab testing company, Wonderland Labs, found 50% of their kratom samples fail lead testing.[5]

How to look for heavy metal testing on a COA

States that have passed the Kratom Consumer Protection Act do not necessarily require that kratom products pass heavy metal testing, so do your homework on brands. While it would be optimal for the kratom COA to report parts per million (ppm) for each of the big four heavy metals (lead, arsenic, cadmium, and mercury), some COAs lump them all together as one "heavy metals" listing.

Your kratom vendor should be able to produce a Certificate of Analysis (COA) that has third-party lab testing for heavy metals printed on it for the batch sold to you or at least within the past 12 months. Remember, the more recent the lab test COA, the more certain you can be that your product is safe.

TESTING FOR ADULTERANTS

Kratom is sometimes tested for adulterants, but it's not often listed on a COA. It is unclear how often kratom products are intentionally adulterated in the grey market, but it is rare to see in trusted kratom vendors that follow good manufacturing practices and provide COAs for testing of other components.[6]

Government agencies like the FDA and research scientists are usually the only ones who run tests to see if kratom product that is supposed to be 100% kratom has fillers in it or added active ingredients to make users feel higher or sleepier. An examples of a relatively innocuous filler is the sugar maltodextrin. Dangerous adulterants that have resulted in potential drug-drug interactions and even death in kratom users include neurotransmitter phenylethylamine (PEA), the synthetic cannabinoid "Spice," opioids, and benzodiazepines.[7]

Adding extra alkaloids to boost potency is not allowed
Interestingly, adding synthetic mitragynine or 7-hydoxymitragynine to any kratom containing product is also considered an adulteration of kratom products.[8] This is because additional alkaloids could cause unexpected adverse effects like increased sleepiness, drug-drug interactions, overdose, and death. Anything kratom powder containing over 2% potency of 7-hydoxymitragynine is considered adulterated, because the plant cannot make any more than that naturally.

Several kratom brands have shown interested in creating enhanced kratom products, similar to how cannabis has lines of super potent cannabis concentrates or terpene-enhanced cannabis products. The American Kratom Association suggests that these kratom brands who want to add extra alkaloids to kratom powder or extracts submit an application to the FDA for a new dietary ingredient (NDI) before marketing or selling such a product.[9] This is a costly and lengthy process, which means these types of products most likely won't be seen legally on the market for years.

In states that have passed the Kratom Consumer Protection Act, it is a crime to knowingly sell adulterated products to consumers, including those with added mitragynine or 7-hydroxymitragynine.[10] Hopefully with more states passing this legislation, adulterated kratom products will be a thing of the past, and kratom will be safe for everyone to use.

TESTING FOR BACTERIA, FUNGI, AND MYCOTOXINS

Kratom can be contaminated with bacteria, yeast, and mold at any point during its growing, harvesting, processing, and packaging.

Kratom is often specifically tested for:

- Presence of salmonella bacteria
- Presence of E. coli bacteria
- Presence of staphylococcus bacteria
- Presence of coliform bacteria
- Aerobic plate count - levels of some bacteria
- Presence of yeast
- Presence of mold

Ingesting kratom with E. coli or other bacteria in it can cause nausea, abdominal cramping, diarrhea, vomiting, gas, fever, and fatigue. Ingesting kratom with yeast or mold can cause many of the same issues as well as allergic reactions in some consumers.

According to Wonderland Labs, a third-party kratom lab

testing site, 5% of their kratom samples failing their aerobic plate counts, 15% have high levels of mold, and a whopping 30% fail for presence of E. coli bacteria.[11] While this sounds awful, remember kratom is a plant-based powder tea that can be easily contaminated by exposure with air, moisture, and the people handling it. That's why testing is so important so unsafe products don't make it to market.

TESTING FOR PESTICIDES

Pesticide testing is usually required for hemp and cannabis products, but it is usually absent from kratom COAs. This is unfortunate, as many patients can be sensitive to the chemicals in pesticides and need to know which ones are used.

Kratom farmers could be using pesticides in their country that are illegal to use in the United States, similar to what we often saw with cannabis products. These illegal pesticides can be especially dangerous if consumed in smokable products or ingested daily. Side effects of these pesticides can include headaches, nausea, diarrhea, vomiting, chest pain, joint pain, and confusion.[12]

What about organic kratom?
Kratom is a cousin of the coffee tree, so it's worth noting that the pesticides used on coffee effect the flavor of the drink. Many people prefer certified organic coffee that is free of chemical pesticides and fertilizers. While kratom can't be certified organic yet because it needs to pass other legal classifications as a food source first, the consumer should be able to know whether their kratom is clean or covered in toxic pesticides.

Hopefully the kratom industry will demand pesticide testing on COAs as the industry matures and set regulations for what are acceptable pesticides and quantity limits. While extra pesticide testing and potential product recalls will obviously make kratom products more expensive for both manufacturers and consumers, ultimately it will make the kratom industry much more safe.

PROPER STORAGE OF KRATOM AT HOME

Kratom safety doesn't stop with the manufacturer. Kratom is sensitive to light, oxygen, and moisture. Once you open up and start using your kratom, it's important that you store it safely to prevent bacteria and mold from growing in it, as well as prevent the active alkaloids from degrading and not working anymore.

Make sure to follow these rules when it comes to storing your kratom:

- Keep your kratom in a dark place like a cabinet and not on your countertop.
- Don't store your kratom in clear bags or jars. If your kratom vendor packaged it with see-through panels, etc, make sure to put the bag inside an opaque bag.
- Keep your kratom dry and do not store it in the fridge.
- Close your container of kratom as soon as possible after you have taken what you need out of it.
- Make sure to squeeze out excess oxygen before zipping up your bag of kratom.
- Divide large bags of kratom into smaller bags and vacuum seal them until you're ready to use them.
- Store large sealed bags of kratom in your freezer until you're ready to use them.
- Don't store your kratom in a cigar humidor or a cannabis humidor. There are different

THE SAFETY PROFILE OF KRATOM

environments that are optimal for storing tobacco, cannabis and kratom.

ACCIDENTAL KRATOM OVERDOSE

If you accidentally ingest much more kratom than you wanted, or your child or pet got into your kratom, make sure to call the Poison Control Center at (800) 222-1222. It's a free hotline available 24/7, and can help you avoid a costly and usually unnecessary trip to the ER.

While respiratory depression from kratom is much less likely to happen than with heroin, morphine and other opioids, it is possible when the user has taken a very high dose of kratom and taken alcohol or other drugs. In some cases, Narcan (naloxone) is necessary to reverse overdose.[13] If you suspect someone has overdosed on kratom and other drugs, call 911 immediately.

KRATOM CAN'T KILL YOU BY ITSELF

There is three main reasons why kratom is unlikely to cause overdose and death by respiratory depression, while other opioids do. Mitragynine and 7-hydroxymitragynine are both only partial agonists of the mu opioid receptor, meaning that they don't activate them 100% like morphine, oxycodone, or fentanyl do.

The main alkaloids in kratom also activate the mu opioid receptor without activating a protein called beta-arrestin. Beta-arrestin is associated with the pathway that causes diaphragm muscles to slow and breathing to stop. So, when kratom activates the mu opioid receptor to relieve pain and boost mood, it does so without the risk of respiratory depression and death.[14]

Finally, both mitragynine and 7-hydroxymitragynine kratom alkaloids are actually antagonists of the delta and kappa opioid receptors, meaning that they are blocking those receptors and slowing down tolerance. This would prevent a user from taking higher doses that could be dangerous.

ARE AMERICANS MORE VULNERABLE TO KRATOM OVERDOSE?

Residents of Thailand and other countries where kratom is grown have consumed it for thousands of years without the severity of the adverse effects we are now seeing in the United States. Cases of using kratom to get high that resulted in calls to 55 poison control centers in the National Poison Data System (NPDS) in the United States and the Ramathibodi Poison Center (RPC) in Thailand from 2010 to 2017 were analyzed.[15]

Researchers found recreational kratom users who reported kratom overdoses to the poison control hotlines from either country were equally likely to use kratom with opioids or benzodiazepines, Americans were more likely to take other sedatives with kratom, and more likely to have severe clinical outcomes. But why?

It's possible that Americans may be using kratom adulterated with unsafe drugs, whereas people in Thailand were getting pure kratom because it was grown there. Another possibility is that Americans are less educated about how to use kratom safely, or that because of extensive prescription drug histories, our livers are less healthy. Perhaps Americans have different versions of opioid receptors that make them more vulnerable to adverse effects of kratom.

KRATOM WILL BE EVEN SAFER TO USE IN THE FUTURE

It's important to understand what is different about kratom products, kratom use, kratom education, and health of kratom users in different parts of the world so we can reduce the harms of using this natural plant medicine.

We also must work to pass the Kratom Consumer Protection Act (KCPA) in more states as well as the federal level to ensure minors don't use kratom and all products are third-party lab tested. Safer products, partnered with harm reduction education as well as reduced stigma of use will lead to kratom being adopted as a safe, plant-based alternative to pain management.

CHAPTER 6

HOW TO USE KRATOM AS MEDICINE

Tea, wine, beer, cannabis, CBD, kratom. What do they all have in common? A learning curve of language used to describe what products are, how they are made, and how they work in your body. Maybe you've mastered all the cannabis terminology and strain names and are shocked to find kratom has its own unique set of strains and definitions. For a new kratom user, this kratom industry language can make choosing and using a kratom product confusing.

This chapter provides an overview of the different ways to use kratom, the future innovation of kratom products, how to pick a kratom strain, kratom dosing, way to avoid building kratom tolerance, and how to use kratom responsibly. By the end of the chapter you should feel confident about which type of product you would like to start out with, how much to take, and what to do if you experience adverse effects.

KRATOM VEINS AND STRAIN NAMES

While some concentrated kratom products, like kratom shots, kratom tinctures, or kratom vapes most likely will not state what strain they are made from, it's important to pick the right

HOW TO USE KRATOM AS MEDICINE

kratom strains when you're using kratom capsules, kratom powder, and kratom tea.

There are four major classes of kratom strains: white vein, red vein, green vein, and yellow vein kratom. Each of these strain classes differ by how the kratom leaves are dried and processed, and have different amounts of alkaloids in them. They also tend to differ in effects, as some can be more energetic while some provide stronger pain relief.

White vein kratom
White vein kratom is known for providing short bursts of energy and focus, making it more similar to your morning coffee than a pain killer or an antidepressant. It is not very euphoric or good at pain relief. White vein kratom is often preferred for morning use or to get through the afternoon slump.

Green vein kratom
For those who find white vein kratom makes them too wired, green vein kratom can provide a more relaxed energy burst, rounded out with a mood lift and mild pain relief. Green vein kratom is great for beginner users.

Red vein kratom
Red vein kratom usually has the highest amount of 7-hydroxymitragynine, the alkaloid that provides the longest and highest amount of pain relief. While some strains provide pain relief and energy at low doses, at moderate to high doses, red vein kratom can relieve pain, increase euphoria, and promote sleep. Red vein kratom is often preferred for nighttime use.

Yellow vein kratom
Yellow vein kratom is actually controversial as a new class of kratom. Some say it is white kratom that is just dried differently, while other say picking the leaf off the plant at a

different time, when different alkaloids are expressed, causes this unique coloring. The effects of yellow vein kratom different from white vein kratom in that yellow vein kratom usually lasts longer, and is more euphoric and pain relieving than white kratom.

Popular kratom strains

Borneo, Bali, Indo, Maenga Da, Malay, Sumatra, and Thai are popular names of kratom. The names are often based on where they are grown, and the environmental conditions change the alkaloid content and effects. Maeng Da strains are famous for their high 7-hydroxymitragynine content and long-lasting effects. Each of these names will be paired with the vein class they are in, so you might see a Red Maeng Da kratom strain and a Green Maeng Da kratom strain, for example.

CHOOSING A KRATOM STRAIN

Finding a kratom strain that's right for you may be easier than finding the perfect cannabis strain to smoke, as there is less than fifty kratom strains, and thousands of cannabis strains. Many kratom consumers keep at least one strain from each class to rotate through to reduce potential kratom tolerance, which is discussed later on in the chapter.

It's important to keep notes so that you know what dose and strains work best for you. When using a new kratom strain, note how how it makes you feel every hour in terms of energy, focus, pain relief, anxiety relief, mood boost, or sleepiness. Make sure to note the dose in grams you took, and whether it was capsules, tea, or toss and wash. Note whether you used kratom on an empty stomach, and if you didn't when your last meal was. Write down any medications you took and when you took them, in case you have any drug-drug interactions

Some strains may make you feel energized as first, and then relax you so much you fall asleep. Every person is different, and you may find a strain that others describe as energetic may make you sleepy or vice versa, especially if you take too low or too high of a dose. Many people find they like low doses of energizing strains in the morning, and higher doses of pain relieving strains in the evening. By taking good notes, you'll find what kratom regimen works best for you.

ROUTES OF ADMINISTRATION

There are many ways to use kratom, but in the United States, the most common is using kratom capsules, swallowing kratom powder, or drinking kratom tea.

Every patient responds differently to kratom, as we have different liver health, digestive health, and brain chemistry. It's important to start low and go slow when it comes to dosing kratom, just like with cannabis. Too much kratom can make you feel ill instead of relief or relaxation.

KRATOM CAPSULES

Kratom capsules are eaten, so they fall under the delivery method category of ingestion. A kratom capsule is a pill containing kratom powder on the inside and a gelatin or cellulose shell on the outside. Gelatin kratom capsules are not vegetarian or vegan, but cellulose capsules are. Be careful if you are allergic to certain food colorings, as some capsules are not clear and contain FD&C food colorings like Yellow #5 or Red #40.

Dosing

For a beginner dose, try using 1 gram of kratom. The capsule size may vary, as well as the density of kratom packed inside them. However, a good starter dose should be 2 capsules, as most capsules contain 1/2 a gram of kratom.

As you become more experienced with kratom, you can increase your dose up to 2.5 grams. Users that have built up tolerance, or those with severe pain, can usually take up to 5 grams without adverse effects. High dose kratom is considered between 5 and 10 grams of kratom.

Absorption
Kratom capsules usually kick in with 30-45 minutes of use, however, certain factors can change how your kratom capsules are digested. Make sure to drink enough water to swallow your capsules, but not too much as it may prevent your kratom from being absorbed. Some users like to drink their capsules with lemon water or orange juice to increase the potency and onset of effects.

Take kratom capsules on empty stomach for the fastest and most complete absorption, as food in your stomach can delay absorption. Take your kratom capsules 45 minutes before a meal or 90 minutes after a meal for best results. The effects of kratom capsules usually last 2-3 hours, and many users dose more than once daily.

KRATOM TABLETS

Kratom tablets also exist, and they are kratom powder that is pressed into a tablet form and do not have a capsule. They are often more expensive than kratom capsules, but have the benefit that there is more kratom per volume and they tend to be smaller and easier to swallow.

Check with the manufacturer to see how many grams of kratom are in each tablet to determine what your dose is for a beginner or experienced kratom user, as it may differ from the number of capsules you have previously taken.

The same rules about eating kratom capsules apply to eating kratom tablets. Kratom tablets may have a slightly faster onset due to a lack of capsule for the stomach to digest.

KRATOM POWDER

Kratom powder can be eaten or added to drinks, so it also falls under the delivery method category of ingestion. Kratom leaves are dried and ground into fine powder that can be added to drinks or foods, put into capsules, or swallowed via a method called toss & wash. Kratom tea is kratom powder added to hot water. Lemon, sugar, and other flavorings are often added to kratom tea to mask the bitter taste. Kratom edibles include kratom gummies, and kratom chocolates.

Similar to chugging a shot of alcohol, the toss and wash method is about getting as much of the gross tasting kratom in your body at once without spending time or money on kratom capsules or using kratom edibles. Some people merely weigh out their kratom and throw it their mouth, washing it down with a drink that masks the flavor. Others package their kratom in a damp tissue before throwing it their mouth to prevent the powders from spreading everywhere or coughing it back up.

Absorption

Kratom tea may be absorbed faster than kratom capsules, kicking in between 10 and 30 minutes. The toss and wash method is one of the fastest ways to absorb kratom, and many users feel effects in 5-10 minutes. The effects of kratom powder or kratom tea can last 2-4 hours at low doses (1-5 grams), and 4-8 hours at higher doses (5 or more grams). Some strains also last longer than others, potentially due to different combinations of minor alkaloids in the strains.

KRATOM SHOTS

Kratom powder or kratom extract dissolved into flavored drink "shots" is now readily available on the commercial market for dosing kratom on the go. It's likely that the effects of kratom drinks will come on faster than taking kratom capsules or kratom teas due to the concentrated extract in them, as well as other ingredients that may enhance absorption. For a beginner user, it's best to avoid kratom shots, as they make you feel dizzy, high, or sleepy.

KRATOM TINCTURES

Kratom tinctures are not as widely used as kratom powder or kratom capsules, but are beginning to emerge on the market. Similar to CBD oil or THC tinctures, the active alkaloids in kratom can be turned into a concentrated extract that is suspended in alcohol and available in a dropper bottle.

Make sure to check that your tincture is a "full-spectrum" tincture contains all the kratom alkaloids and other chemicals. Otherwise, some tinctures are just mitragynine extracts in alcohol or oil and will be less effective, or worse, potentially dangerous because they are too concentrated.

The liquid is dropped under the tongue and held for 30 seconds, where it absorbed sublingually and enters the bloodstream within 10-15 minutes. Sublingual administration avoids the gut and liver, making a potent way to deliver kratom for those who are having problems with bioavailability. It is also one of the least studied methods of using kratom, and may put users at higher risk for addiction or unwanted side effects.

INHALATION

Opioids have been smoked for thousands of years, beginning with opium, then heroin, and now kratom. Kratom leaves can also be smoked, and kratom powder can be smoked in pipes. Some people even sprinkle kratom powder on tobacco or cannabis and then smoke it, potentially increasing harms. Smoking kratom may expose the lungs to high amounts of tar, similar to tobacco smoke or cannabis smoke, and may contribute to asthma, COPD, and even lung cancer. Unfortunately, while research studies have determined the chemical makeup of cannabis smoke, no similar studies have been done with kratom smoke.

Kratom vapes have appeared on the market, often sold in the same headshops selling unregulated CBD vapes or bongs for smoking marijuana. It is unclear whether vaping kratom extract is more safe or less safe than smoking kratom leaf. Smoking and vaping kratom is not common compared to the millions of users consuming kratom powder, but is of particular concern because smoking kratom will lead to faster onset, and potentially higher addiction risk.

There is clearly much research needed on the short-term and long-term effects of smoking and vaping kratom. It is strongly suggested that consumers do not smoke or vape kratom, especially since these products are unregulated and it is unclear if adulterants could cause further harm.

CHEWING KRATOM LEAVES

In Thailand many people chew on kratom leaves regularly for energy and pain relief, spitting out the excess plant matter. This is similar to ancient Peruvians chewing coca leaves to release small amounts of cocaine for energy while working, or Americans use chewing tobacco for energy from nicotine.[1] A recent study of people in Thailand who chew kratom leaves regularly found they were more likely to perceive kratom as medicine than non-users who viewed kratom users as drug addicts.[2] This is similar to data on cannabis users, who are less likely to view their consumption as harmful compared to nonusers. It is unclear if chewing kratom leaves comes with any risks. For example, chewing tobacco is associated with increased risk of mouth, tongue, cheek, throat, esophagus, and pancreatic cancer.[3]

TOPICAL APPLICATION

Endogenous opioids and opioid receptors are found in the skin, including in nerve fibers that sense pain and temperature, hair follicles, immune cells, and skin cells including keratinocytes and melanocytes.[4] As the skin can easily become cut or stressed or due to friction, sunburn, or chemical irritation, opioids provide pain relief, and are important for wound repair. Adding kratom to pain relief creams, skincare, bath bombs, and more could be a game changer for patients who are looking for natural ways to look and feel good.

Kratom pain relief creams

Topical opioids are being looked at as an alternative to prescription opioid pills for pain management. Typically they are produced at compounding pharmacies by converting opioid pills into opioid creams or lotions for localized pain relief. Out of all the topical applications for kratom, kratom as a pain relief cream with anti-inflammatory properties is most promising.

Kratom has been used traditionally as a wound poultice.[5] Because kratom alkaloids are weaker that prescription opioids when used topically, it is likely that kratom pain relief creams may provide mild but long-lasting pain relief. Homemade kratom pain relief lotion or pain balm may be more effective when combined with ingredients that provide pain relief, such as peppermint, eucalyptus, lavender, frankincense oil, or CBD oil.

Kratom lotion may also be more effective at pain relief if combined with lidocaine. Research suggests low dose lidocaine combined with a low morphine topical are more effective together for pain relief than the effects of both by themselves.[6] A kratom and lidocaine topical lotion could be effective for sunburn pain as well as neuropathic pain.

Kratom skincare
Kratom contains alkaloids and flavonoids that have antioxidant, antinflammatory, antibacterial, and even anticancer properties, and have been used topically in traditional Thai medicine for skin conditions.[7] This means kratom-infused beauty products may have an enhanced ability to fight acne or skin aging, but no clinical research studies have proven that. There may be utility in adding kratom into sunscreens or face creams if it helps prevent growth of skin cancer cells.[8]

Kratom acts differently when applied topically to your skin than used internally. Some people report increased acne when eating kratom daily, especially if they were prone to it before starting kratom consumption. If eating kratom is causing cystic acne, discontinue use.

Kratom soap
There are recipes online for making your own kratom soap from extra kratom powder you have at home and some people are even selling homemade kratom soap. But is it worth it? Kratom soap appears to have no extra benefits

over regular soap and is a good way to waste kratom medicine.

While some manufacturers have promoted kratom soap as a way to stop itchy skin, it's likely a false claim. Opioids, whether taken internally or applied topically, often result in increased itchiness as a side effect. In fact, opioid antagonists that block opioid receptors in the skin are used to treat dry, itchy skin and conditions like atopic dermatitis.[9,10]

Kratom bath bombs
CBD and cannabis have exploded as topicals for the bath tub, with infused bath bombs and epsom bath salts being very popular for pain relief, muscle tension, and relaxation. But are kratom bath bombs or kratom bath salts a thing? And do they work?

Similar to CBD and cannabis topicals, it is unlikely that kratom topicals can be absorbed through the skin into the bloodstream to cause a high. The skin does have opioid receptors, and soaking in a hot bath with a kratom bath bomb may help reduce nerve pain and muscle tension.

This method of using kratom is not well researched, and it is not clear how effective it is compared to CBD or THC bath bombs. While results may not be super impressive compared to other pain relievers added to the bath like peppermint oil or eucalyptus oil, it certainly shouldn't cause harm.

Kratom bath salts
It's hard to do a search for kratom bath salts, because instead of kratom-infused Epsom salts popping up on your Google search, comparisons of kratom to "bath salts" a recreational stimulant containing concentrated chemicals from the khat

plant, such as methylenedioxypyrovalerone (MDPV), mephedrone and methylone.[11]

It's likely using kratom bath salts will have many of the same benefits as using kratom bath bombs, with the added bonus of muscle relaxation from the magnesium sulfate in the Epsom salts. Try mixing some kratom powder with Epsom salts and throw them in your bath to see if it works for you.

KRATOM TRANSDERMAL PENS AND PATCHES

Topical lotions can turn into transdermal lotions that do enter the bloodstream depending on where they are applied and whether ingredients that help topicals penetrate the skin more deeply. In the cannabis industry, CBD and THC transdermal gel pens sold by companies like Mary's Medicinals and Nanosphere Health Sciences are applied to the wrist for consistent, fast microdosing of cannabinoids for pain relief without having to smoke marijuana or swallow pills.

Transdermal opioids are already on the market
Are kratom transdermal pens or patches even possible as a product? Transdermal opioid patches are used in medicine for pain management and are safer, more effective, and have less adverse side effects that oral morphine.[12]

Opioid transdermal patches include fentanyl patches and buprenorphine patches, which are highly effective for both cancer pain and neuropathic pain. Buprenorphine is very interesting because it is a synthetic opioid that is similar to mitragynine in being a partial MOR agonist and antagonist at KOR and DOR. It is possible that kratom alkaloids could be used transdermally for moderate to severe pain in the same way.

Advantages of transdermal kratom

Why would someone want to use a kratom transdermal pen over other products? The amount of kratom capsules needed to be swallowed for a patient with severe pain can be 5 or more several times a day. For patients with medical conditions like multiple sclerosis or fibromyalgia, swallowing may be difficult.

Kratom also has a very bitter taste when eaten or drank, or used as a sublingual, and unlike cannabis, is not commonly smoked. For patients looking to use kratom for pain relief on the go, it requires having a drink to swallow pills or make tea with. It's not convenient. For these patients, a quick swipe of a transdermal gel pen on the wrist would be a discrete way to relieve pain without the hassle of drinking nasty tasting kratom powder or swallowing handfuls of capsules.

Enhanced bioavailability of transdermal kratom

Biovailability of kratom alkaloids is low when eaten, and kratom is subject to first-pass metabolism in the liver. This means patients looking for pain management may have to eat kratom several times a day for relief. Transdermal application of opioids allows for consistent blood levels of opioids and long-lasting pain relief.[13] Kratom transdermal patches or pens would also avoid first-pass metabolism in the liver, meaning lower doses of kratom alkaloids could be used, reducing potential adverse effects.

Disadvantages of transdermal opioids

It can take 24 hours for blood levels of opioids from a transdermal patch or gel pen to reach levels sufficient for pain relief after first use. For the general population of kratom users, this is manageable, but for users who are in recovery from heroin and opioid dependent, withdrawal symptoms could be experienced during that time.

Another disadvantage is that it can take a day or longer for opioids to clear the bloodstream once blood levels are stable. This can be problematic if there are any adverse side effects like nausea or respiratory depression, and may require Narcan administration to reverse. While kratom has fewer adverse side effects than stronger opioids, they still occur.

Are kratom transdermal pens and patches the future?
It is unclear if kratom transdermal products will be sold by kratom manufacturers or developed into single alkaloid transdermal products like a 7-hydroxymitragynine transdermal patch by pharmaceutical companies. I do not recommend trying to create your own kratom transdermal patches and pens at home, as much research is required to make sure this new delivery method is safe. We are likely at least 5 years from commercially produced kratom transdermal products.

RECTAL SUPPOSITORIES

Almost any prescription medication can be transformed into a rectal suppository by a compounding pharmacy, and this includes opioid medications. One commonly used rectal suppository, B & O Supprettes, is a combination of belladonna and opium used to relieve pain and reduce use of opioids before or after urinary, prostate, or vaginal surgeries.[14,15]

Suppositories aren't just limited to prescription medications, as many people purchase or make their suppositories using herbal preparations of ingredients like garlic or essential oils. Cannabis suppositories are available commercially by companies like FORIA Wellness, and are used for relief of back, pelvic, and gut pain. While there has been anecdotal evidence for the benefits and safety of cannabis rectal suppositories, there is limited research published. While kratom suppositories aren't available yet commercially, it is unclear whether they are safe or effective for any form of pain. Perhaps like with cannabis suppositories, there is the taboo of rectal administration to get over. The likely possibility is that the risk of overdose make experimentation too risky. At this time we do not recommend making or using kratom suppositories at home. We do support research into this innovative route of administration for relief of severe pelvic or back pain.

INCREASE IN KRATOM USE LEADS TO INCREASE IN REPORTED ADVERSE EFFECTS

Drugs tend to be used and abused at a higher rate in the United States than other countries, especially when it comes to opioids. While there has been a steady increase in reports of adverse effects of kratom and kratom overdoses, there has also been more awareness of kratom as a pain management and prescription opioid substitution. More users of any unfamiliar drug equals more adverse effects. For example, in Colorado, two studies found that ER visits for marijuana overdoses initially spiked and returned to normal the year or two after two events: legalization of medical marijuana, and legalization of recreational marijuana.[16,17] Education on proper dosing and harm reduction, as well as the passage of time, will minimize this temporary spike in kratom accidents.

ADVERSE SIDE EFFECTS

Kratom, like any drug, can cause side effects ranging from mild to severe in some users. Common side effects include:

- Drowsiness
- Nausea
- Constipation
- Dry mouth
- Headache
- Anxiety

Serious side effects include:

- Dizziness
- Vomiting
- Breathing issues
- Seizure

KRATOM NAUSEA

Nausea is a common symptom with many causes, but for kratom users, kratom nausea is especially common side effect. It's usually just a brief and unpleasant experience, but sometimes it can be chronic and serious.

Kratom is used by millions of people around the world for energy, relaxation, and pain relief, but that doesn't mean it doesn't have unwanted side effects in some users. Like any substance, it's important to use kratom responsibly, listen to your body, treat normal side effects, and know when to get help if something is seriously wrong.

Ways to get rid of kratom nausea fast:

1. Take a low dose of kratom the first time using it.
You're most likely to experience nausea, stomach pains, or even vomiting the first time you take kratom, especially if you take a very high dose. A low dose can mean 1 capsule of kratom or 1/2 a teaspoon of kratom powder. Remember many substances, from cannabis, to prescription drugs, have the most powerful unwanted side effects the first day or two you use them as your body adjusts.

2. Make sure to use the lowest dose of kratom that works for you.
The higher the kratom dose, the more likely kratom nausea may happen. Kratom tends to promote relaxation and sleep at higher doses than lower doses. If you are using kratom before bed and feeling nauseous, it might be time to think about using other remedies for sleep instead, like CBD or chamomile tea.

3. Take kratom breaks.
Daily use of kratom may irritate your stomach lining if you are sensitive, and can also contribute to kratom tolerance, where you need higher and higher doses to get the same effects. Taking 1-2 day breaks for even a week long break can help reset your kratom tolerance and help your gut heal.

4. Don't eat kratom on an empty stomach.
Kratom is more easily absorbed on an empty stomach whether in capsule or tea form. That means your usual dose could feel stronger and cause more unwanted side effects like nausea if you haven't eaten in a long time. New users are especially discouraged from using kratom on an empty stomach.

HOW TO USE KRATOM AS MEDICINE

5. Sip on kratom tea slowly.
Don't use the "toss and wash" method of taking kratom powder all at once like a shot of alcohol and washing it down with a drink.

6. Chew on ginger.
Candied ginger and crushed ginger paste are both sweet and spicy and highly effective for reducing nausea fast. If eating is too much for you, try sipping on ginger tea.

7. Eat light.
Choose bland foods like crackers and bananas. Skip anything greasy or spicy. It may also help to eat smaller and more frequent meals and snacks.

8. Drink water.
Stay hydrated with clear fluids including plain water or diluted broth and juice. Take a break from caffeinated beverages such as coffee, tea, and colas.

9. Limit alcohol.
Drinking too much irritates your stomach lining and causes acids to build up. If you find it difficult to use alcohol in moderation, talk with your doctor or call a helpline to find out what resources are available in your area.

10. Avoid strong smells.
You may be sensitive to certain odors, especially if you're pregnant. For relief, try cold foods and fresh air. Don't use kratom if you are pregnant or breastfeeding.

11. Rinse your mouth.
What if you've already eaten something that doesn't agree with you? Take a sip of cold water and swish it around to wash away the residue.

12. Slow down.
Any movement can make you feel more uncomfortable when your stomach is uneasy, so be quiet and sit still. Eating and drinking at a more leisurely pace can help prevent nausea too.

13. Prepare for travel as a kratom user.
You're less likely to experience motion sickness if you face forward during car rides or book a cabin in the middle of a ship. Keep your eyes straight ahead instead of looking at a screen or a book.

14. Know when it's an emergency.
If your nausea and vomiting symptoms are severe, you are on multiple medications, or you accidentally took way too much kratom and are worried about a kratom overdose, please call your doctor immediately or go to the ER. While most kratom users have no issues, kratom is not right for everyone, and some users may have adverse reactions that require hospital treatment.[18]

See your doctor if nausea lasts for more than a few days or you have any additional symptoms that you're concerned about. Otherwise, you can minimize nausea by identifying your own personal triggers and consuming bland foods or clear liquids when you start to feel uncomfortable.

Experiencing nausea or vomiting from kratom use as an experienced user can be a sign that you are using too much kratom or using it too frequently, which can lead to kratom abuse and kratom addiction. Please contact a free substance abuse hotline if you are worried you might be abusing kratom.

KRATOM TOLERANCE

Maybe you're curious about the best way to take kratom powder but scared you might get addicted to it. Or maybe you're an experienced user who is worried they are spending too much money on kratom and getting less and less effects every day. If you're a CBD user or cannabis user, you're familiar with tolerance to cannabis products with daily use. Something very similar happens with regular kratom use, often faster than with cannabis.

What is kratom tolerance?

Kratom tolerance is real, and unchecked, it can lead to kratom dependence, and even worse kratom addiction. But before you get too scared, remember that most people have built up tolerance to caffeine and in fact, are slightly addicted to their daily cup (or two or three) of coffee. Since kratom is actually part of the coffee family of plants, keep in mind kratom dependence is more like caffeine addiction and less like heroin addiction.

How does kratom tolerance form?

The alkaloids in kratom, including mitragynine and 7-hydroxymitragynine, bind to mu and delta opioid receptors on cells and activate downstream pathways that result in effects like pain relief and euphoria. With chronic use of kratom, the opioid receptors become densensitized to the alkaloids, and the downstream pathways are less likely to be turned on. This means a reduction in effects pain relief and mood lift, or the feeling that the kratom isn't working any more.

WAYS TO PREVENT KRATOM TOLERANCE

Reducing your kratom tolerance can require some changes to your daily kratom use, but it doesn't have to involve quitting kratom for good.

Don't use kratom powder every day
The more often you take kratom powder, the faster you will build tolerance to it. There is two ways to reduce frequency of kratom use: how many days per week you use it, and how many times per day you use it.

Consider using kratom powder every other day or two days on, one day off to keep your receptors sensitive to kratom and reduce kratom tolerance. As a beginner user, don't use kratom more than once a day. More experienced kratom users or those who need substantial relief may use kratom no more than twice a day.

Use small doses of kratom powder
As a new user, start low with your dosage. While each brand and even strain of kratom may weight slightly different, the average weight of 1 teaspoon of kratom powder at AURA Therapeutics is about 2.4 grams.

Anything that feels good is best in moderation. Think of that nightly glass of wine that turns into nightly bottle of wine over time. It's best not to make relaxing with a cup of kratom tea a daily habit that turns into 2 or 3 cups. Catch yourself if you find your use growing in time or signs that you're consuming for no other reason except boredom.

Rotate kratom strains
Are you using your favorite kratom strain daily? You may find switching to a different strain may help your body respond

better to the same dose of kratom. For best effects, pick a strain in a different family and alternate use. We recommend have at least one red vein kratom powder, green vein kratom powder, and white vein kratom powder at hand to rotate between.

Why does your body build tolerance to a specific strain? This effect is called Stagnant Strain Syndrome. It's very similar to how cannabis users find they have to switch up the cannabis strains they smoke so they don't have escalate their dose to feel the same effects. Cannabis contains over 100 cannabinoids, terpenes, and flavonoids, each with their own combination in individual strains.

Different strains of kratom contains different levels and combinations of active ingredients including 40 alkaloids such as mitragynine and 7-hydroxymitragynine, flavonoids, polyphenols, and terpenoid saponins. While we are still learning about the different chemical profiles of individual strains, we do know that they may activate opioid and other receptors differently and result in less tolerance when more than one is used regularly.

Use kratom potentiators instead of more kratom powder
It's tempting to think more is always better, but in the case of kratom, you can use less kratom if you combine it with other natural plant substances that potentiate its effects. For example, add a bit of lemon juice to your kratom powder and the citric acid will help break down plant material and release the active alkaloids more quickly. Many users report taking a magnesium capsule improves the effects of using kratom, likely because most people are deficient in magnesium to begin with.

Some natural plants inhibit p450 liver enzymes that break

down the active ingredients in kratom, which increase the amount of time they are working in your bloodstream. Grapefruit juice is a known kratom potentiator, but you probably didn't know that CBD also is because it inhibits the CYP3A4 enzyme that breaks down mitragynine. Taking CBD either 45 minutes before kratom use or together in the same tea means you should be able to use less kratom for the same effects. We love using CBD sugar with kratom tea.

Take kratom tolerance breaks

Many CBD and cannabis users find taking a week off resets their tolerance levels. Similarly, taking occasional week or longer kratom tolerance breaks can help your opioid receptors respond better to chronic kratom use.

KRATOM WITHDRAWAL SYNDROME

Users who are dependent or addicted to kratom can experience withdrawal symptoms. They include:

- Muscle aches
- Insomnia
- Irritability
- Aggression
- Mood changes
- Runny nose
- Tremors

Kratom withdrawal symptoms will be worse when the user has regularly consumed very high amounts of kratom and then quit cold turkey. In these patients, kratom withdrawal may appear similar to opioid withdrawal syndrome, and some patients have experienced hallucinations, seizures or other serious effects of withdrawal. Please consult a doctor or ER if you experience severe kratom withdrawal symptoms.

For easing mild kratom withdrawal symptoms, there are some natural options. One cannabinoid in hemp and cannabis, called CBD, has been shown to be effective for opioid withdrawal in clinical studies. CBD oil can be purchased over the counter online or in stores, and is non-addictive. It works to boost mood, reduce insomnia, relieve mild pain, and rebalance receptors during withdrawal.

Taking CBD oil or smoking a marijuana joint could be helpful in relieving mild kratom withdrawal symptoms. Both CBD and THC, the active ingredient in psychoactive strains of cannabis, can modulate how mu and delta opioid receptors respond to opioids as allosteric modulators.[19]

KRATOM ADDICTION

Kratom addiction is characterized in the same was as other substance abuse disorders: compulsive drug taking and drug seeking, inability to control how much one takes, and cravings when access to the drug is limited. If you are worried about your kratom use, please speak with your doctor, or consult a substance abuse hotline, which is listed in the Resources section of this book.

Is kratom rewarding?

A drug has to be rewarding, or pleasurable, for it to be addictive. One test of whether a drug can be abused is intracranial self-stimulation (ICSS), where rodents press a lever to receive an electrical shock to a part of their brain that results in pleasure. Drugs like morphine that have abuse potential will decrease the threshold for ICSS responding. Kratom alkaloids mitragynine and 7-OH-mitragynine did the opposite, showing they do not have abuse potential in this model.[20]

Another study of mitragynine extract in rodents found no

evidence of changes within the mesolimibic pathway, indicating a lack of addiction potential. Rats won't self-administer mitragynine or other kratom alkaloids, but they will self-administer 7-hydroxymitragynine, suggesting that kratom alkaloid that is potentially addictive, if any, would be 7-hydroxymitragynine.[21]

USING KRATOM RESPONSIBLY IS THE MOST IMPORTANT THING YOU CAN DO

Whether you're just starting to use kratom or a longtime user of kratom, it's important to use kratom responsibly so you minimize any unwanted side effects. Remember to listen to your mind and your body and keep your kratom use in moderation.

Just because something is a plant or is natural, does not mean it is automatically safe. This is especially true of anything that might be used daily or at high doses. People can get stomach aches, heart palpitations, and insomnia from drinking too much coffee. People have even died from drinking too much water, which is crazy considering our bodies contain almost 70% water!

If kratom is right for you now, it doesn't mean it will always be right for you. Patients that have had their antidepressant work for years may suddenly need to switch to a new brand, or chronic pain patients need to switch opioids because their tolerance is escalating their dose to dangerous levels. I would rather see a patient switch to another pain management method than escalate their kratom dose to the point where they are having withdrawal symptoms or other dangerous side effects.

By following the tips above to use kratom responsibly, you're making a smart decision about your health. Kratom can be used safely to improve the quality of your life, whether it's to relax or reclaim your energy.

CHAPTER 7
MEDICAL RISKS OF KRATOM USE

Kratom, just like any other supplement, food, or medication, is not right for everyone. It's important to review factors like your current medications, liver and heart health, history of substance abuse, age, and whether or not you are looking to get pregnant before starting kratom. If you want to be more confident you are making the right choice, talk with your physician or an experienced clinician about both the risks and benefits of using kratom for you.

While the media has created hype around kratom being dangerous and addictive, the science says otherwise. If you do experience adverse side effects from using kratom, it's important to know the difference between serious side effects that warrant immediate cessation of use and a potential doctor or ER visit, and ones that are less serious. Most mild side effects experienced with kratom can be reduced by changing delivery method, strains, brand, time of use, or other variables.

DRUG-DRUG INTERACTIONS

Kratom can inhibit many types of p450 liver enzymes that break down medications and drugs in the body. These include CYP2C9, CYP2D6, CYP1A2, and CYP3A4, which accounts for almost all drugs metabolized through the liver. It is currently unclear how clinically relevant kratom's effects are, but a research study at Washington State University is performing a first of its kind drug interaction liability study of kratom.[1]

Worthwhile noting is that calls to poison control centers involving kratom increased 52 times from 2011 to 2017, and one-third of calls were about kratom users who had also taken other medications or drugs including opioids and benzodiazepines.

Most opioids are broken down by the CYP2D6 and CYP3A4 enzymes that kratom inhibits, causing blood levels of these drugs to accumulate, potentially causing respiratory depression while sleep and death. If you are taking opioids or benzodiazepines like Xanax, I strongly caution against using kratom, and suggest CBD oil or cannabis products as a potentially safer alternative.

Mitragynine, the most abundant alkaloid in kratom, was thought to works better to block CYP2D6 liver enzymes than CYP2C9 or CYP3A4 liver enzymes. However, a recent study shows it may increase the length of time drugs metabolized by the CYP3A4 enzymes are in your system by 5.7 times.[2] Other alkaloids in kratom, including paynantheine and corynantheidine, are also known to inhibit CYP2D6 and CYP3A4 enzymes.[3]

Patients that are considering using kratom for long-term pain management should check to see if they are using a medication that is metabolized by CYP2D6 or CYP3A4. If they are, they should talk to their doctor before using kratom or monitor their health closely when using kratom for adverse side effects from a potential drug-drug interaction.

MOST KRATOM USERS DON'T WANT TO BE HIGH

It's important to point out that there are three groups of kratom consumers: those who use kratom as medicine to relieve symptoms, those who are in recovery from opioid abuse, and those who use it recreationally to get high.

The percentage who use it medicinally it is the vast majority, while those who use kratom recreationally are less than 5%. In fact, a survey of 6,150 kratom users run by the Pain News Network found only 1.6% were using kratom for the primary purpose of getting high.[4] This is is opposition to cannabis, where we do see a thriving market of recreational marijuana users in addition to those who consume it for medical reasons.

USERS IN OPIOID RECOVERY MOST AT RISK FOR HARM

Most harms of kratom use are magnified with chronic use of high doses. Recreational kratom users may use higher doses, but are likely only occasionally using it, and are less likely to respond to education about harms of high doses. Medical users of kratom tend to use frequently but at moderate doses to control symptoms. Education aimed at medical users of kratom should be focused on reducing tolerance and preventing escalation of dose.

Kratom users who are coming off of heroin or prescription opioids are the most likely to use high doses of kratom daily, as they are tolerant to the effects of opioids and looking to avoid opioid withdrawal. They are likely to suffer the most adverse side effects of kratom. However, we must balance that with the harm reduction approach of what the worse harms of using heroin and other opioids could be.

Heroin use is associated with a high rate of overdose and death, while kratom is not. Education aimed at opioid dependent kratom users should focus on taking kratom tolerance breaks, lowering dose over time, and stress management.

ACUTE TOXICITY AND OVERDOSE

Adverse effects can happen any time a user uses kratom, especially if it is their first time or they use too high of a dose. The most common adverse effects include nausea, stomach upset, and vomiting. In one case of vomiting that wouldn't stop in a senior using kratom for the first time for joint pain, the patient was admitted to the ER.[5]

In one extreme case, a kratom-naive 15 year old girl consumed 45 x 500 mg kratom capsules at once in a suicide attempt.[6] This 22 g kratom overdose for a child resulted in nausea, vomiting, dizziness, heart palpitations and racing heartbeat, tremors, constricted pupils, and dry mouth. While she was monitored for seizures or cardiac events in the hospital, she did not have any and 14 hours after the kratom overdose she fully recovered. This case clearly shows it difficult to die from kratom if there are no other drugs in your system, and even with an accidental or intentional overdose, there are is long-lasting damage.

LIVER TOXICITY

According to the US Drug Induced Liver Injury Network, there have eleven cases of livery injury after kratom use in the United States requiring hospitalization but not resulting in death.[7] These kratom users were only take kratom for about 14 days before symptoms of jaundice and liver injury appeared, but the average dose was high at 14-21 g of kratom per day. Several users had a current or past history of heavy alcohol or opioid use, suggesting that the liver was not healthy prior to using kratom. The findings of this paper, published in the journal of Drug and Alcohol Dependence, suggests that patients with a history of alcohol, opioid, or benzodiazepine abuse should check whether their liver is healthy enough to take kratom before starting use, and to use the lowest dose possible.

CHRONIC TOXICITY

While the media have demonized kratom use as unsafe, published research suggests long-term harms of kratom cannot be separated from the other recreational and prescription drugs used by patients. In some cases, patients also used kratom that was not lab tested and in fact contained adulterants like synthetic marijuana that cause acute and chronic toxicity. More research is required to access the long-term risks and benefits of using kratom long-term at normal doses.

INCREASED RISK OF ERECTILE DYSFUNCTION

Long-term use of all opioids is associated with higher risk of erectile dysfunction (ED), and at younger ages than expected. 42% of men on methadone or buprenorphine report not being able to achieve or maintain an erection.[8] While no studies have specifically looked at kratom and ED, it's likely that long-term kratom use could mildly increase risk of ED. There is a case report of a man who had reduced testosterone levels and loss of sex drive after consuming kratom regularly and recovered completely two months after stopping kratom use.[9]

LOW CARDIOVASCULAR RISK ASSOCIATED WITH KRATOM USE

It is unclear whether lab research looking at activity of alkaloids in kratom translates to real life harms in human kratom users. A recent in vitro study found mitragynine, the main alkaloid in kratom, may alter potassium channels in the heart, potentially leading to deadly cardiac arrhythmias, or heartbeat irregularities.[10] Another study found kratom alkaloid paynantheine also altered potassium channel function.[11] Contradicting this is a recent study of 100 kratom users and 100 people who did not use kratom that found no difference in heartbeat or heart health as measured by electrocardiogram (ECG).[12]

LOW SEIZURE RISK ASSOCIATED WITH KRATOM USE

There have been three reported cases of seizures associated with kratom use. Since there are millions of kratom users in the United States alone, this suggest the risk of seizure with kratom use is very low. Patients with epilepsy and other seizure disorders are strongly suggested to avoid opioids such as kratom because they lower their seizure threshold.[13]

There is one case of a 27 hear old patient with a history of ADHD, anxiety, and substance abuse having a tonic-clonic seizure after using high doses of kratom for 1 and ½ years.[14] It is unclear whether the seizure activity was due to the high doses of kratom, past medical history, or was just random. We do know that high doses of other opioids, such as heroin, can cause seizures in healthy patients.

Another male patient, age 19, experienced recurrent seizures after using dangerously high amounts of kratom capsules daily for several months to treat anxiety.[15] Seizures stopped when kratom was discontinued and came back when the patient relapsed on kratom. It is unclear whether impurities in the kratom, the patient genetics, an undiagnosed medical condition, or another variable is the cause of this patient's seizures.

USING KRATOM WHILE PREGNANT

The use of any supplement, medication, or drug is not recommended while pregnant or breastfeeding, because of lack of research on potential harm to your child's developing brain and body. This includes kratom, as it is difficult to perform any rigorous studies of kratom or any drug on pregnant women due to ethics boards.

It's not clear if alkaloids in kratom pass through the placenta from mother to baby. We do know other drugs, including heroin, morphine, methadone, and THC in cannabis do cross the placenta, so it's likely kratom alkaloids do too. This means it is expected that kratom alkaloids, at some level, can bind to opioid receptors in your baby's spinal cord and brain.

Neonatal abstinence syndrome
Neonatal abstinence syndrome (NAS) is commonly seen in babies born to mothers who used heroin, prescription opioids, other non-stimulant drugs during pregnancy. Not all babies will experience the same symptoms, as it is dependent on the type and total amount of drug the baby was exposed to.

Signs of NAS include:

- shaking, twitching, or seizures
- rapid or troubled breathing
- excessive crying
- excessive yawning
- vomiting or diarrhea
- trouble sleeping

- fever
- sweaty or blotchy skin
- rigid muscles
- stuffy nose or sneezing[16]

When hospitals encounter babies with NAS symptoms, the gold standard is to treat them with decreasing doses of morphine until they are weaned off of opioids. This obviously has harms to the child, but less than going through potentially deadly withdrawal symptoms.

Increasing cases of NAS are seen with women who have been using kratom, which unlike other opioids, does not show up on a typical urine drug testing screen. But is the NAS truly from kratom?

In most NAS cases, the mother was using ridiculous large amounts of kratom or wasn't just using kratom.[17] Mothers were using other medications, including benzodiazepines, neuroleptics like gabapentin, and cigarettes.[18,19] These drugs also can cause low birth weight or neonatal withdrawal symptoms. Combining these drugs with kratom can cause drug-drug interactions that may be even more detrimental to the fetus.

Other possible negative birth outcomes

Kratom use during pregnancy may cause other complications even if NAS is not experienced by your child. Studies of children born to mothers who used other opioids like heroin or morphine experienced stillbirth, low birth weight, preterm delivery, and increase cesarean section delivery.[20] Because kratom alkaloids are less potent that other opioids, it is possible that these pregnancy outcomes will be less severe or nonexistent in kratom users. Birth defects with opioids are not reported, and are not expected with kratom use.

MEDICAL RISKS OF KRATOM USE

Supporting pregnant mothers who use kratom

It is not clear whether using kratom at low doses during pregnancy results in NAS or other negative pregnancy outcomes. It's important to not pass judgement on mothers who use kratom, as many mothers are not healthy before they get pregnant. Some mothers have chronic pain conditions like fibromyalgia, and have to make calculated decisions on whether opioids or kratom are safer during pregnancy. For these moms, kratom may be the safer option, and should be counseled on harm reduction.

As a healthcare provider, you may be angry if you find your patient is trying to hide their kratom use from you. Remember that mothers are afraid their healthcare provider will call Child Protective Services (CPS) and take their child away from them for being a negligent mother. Anecdotally, there are thousands of mothers, many with chronic illness, who have used kratom during pregnancy with mild if any withdrawal symptoms seen in their babies.[21] Ask yourself if calling CPS on a kratom using mother is the right thing to do before you do so.

USING KRATOM WHILE BREASTFEEDING

There is even less research on using kratom while breastfeeding than there is on mothers using kratom while pregnant. We have to assume mothers breastfeeding while using kratom were also using kratom while pregnant. Research shows other opioids as well as THC and CBD pass through breastmilk, so it is assumed that kratom alkaloids will be as well.[22]

Breastfeeding mothers are often prescribed opioids by their doctors to handle pain after labor or cesarean section delivery. While opioid exposure in newborns through breastmilk is considered low risk, mothers and healthcare professionals are cautioned to looking for changes in feeding, constipation, and excessive sleepiness that may suggest the baby is more sensitive than normal to opioids. Doctors also suggest women who are taking the most common opioid prescribed, Percocet, which is a combination of oxycodone and acetaminophen, "pump and dump" is they are taking more than 40 mg of oxycodone a day.[23]

What can we learn from this? If you have to use kratom while breastfeeding, try to use the lowest dose possible as infrequently as you can. If you can't lower your dose, make sure to breastfeed first, then take your kratom. If you can't avoid consuming large doses of kratom, consider the "pump and dump" method or potentially switching to infant formula.

RISKS OF CHILDREN USING KRATOM

There are currently no guidelines for the use of opioids for pain management in children, despite their widespread use and potential for addiction, overdose, and death. Prescription opioids fentanyl, morphine, and methadone have been FDA approved for use at all ages, including newborns, while oxycodone and hydromorphone are approved for over the age of 6 months of age and hydrodocone is often used for patients under the age of 2.[24]

Sadly, there has been little research on what the effects of acute or chronic exposure on the developing brain. My work studying the effects of drugs such on heroin on adult neurogenesis, which is the birth of new brain cells in the hippocampus of the adult brain, suggest opioids decrease it. It is likely opioids can also slow brain cell growth in children or teens, and that may include kratom alkaloids.

Many states have made it illegal to sell kratom to adults under 21 or minors under 18, but that doesn't necessarily criminalize their use. At what age is kratom an appropriate alternative for prescription opioids in children or teens with chronic pain? Misuse of prescription opioids among teens was 8% back in 2015 and is likely to be much higher now.[25] Because kratom alkaloids do not active beta-arresting and do not activate respiratory depression, they may be a safer bet for teenagers who may consume their medications in less responsible ways than adults.

Do not let your child or teen consume kratom recreationally. Until we know more about kratom and its safety in children and teens, your best bet is to avoid letting your child use it unless they have severe chronic pain or are fighting an addiction to heroin or prescription opioid pills. In either case, it's important to have an open conversation with your child's healthcare provider and run tests to make sure their liver and general health is optimal.

RISKS OF DRIVING UNDER THE INFLUENCE OF KRATOM

Kratom can have a wide range effects, from providing energy and focus to causing euphoria and sleepiness. These effects are dependent on the strains used as well as the amounts. Smaller amounts of kratom are likelier to cause less impairment than higher doses. Never drive if you feel too sleepy to pay attention to the road.

There have been instances of kratom being in the bloodstream of deadly crashes. In one case, a toxicology screen revealed a drunk driver who killed a child had kratom in her system, as well as alcohol and fentanyl. Because alcohol, opioids, benzodiazepines, and sedatives can increase the euphoric and sedative effects of kratom, do not drive while using kratom and these substances. To learn more about the legal risks of driving while using or possessing kratom, see the Appendix.

SUMMARY

Kratom is most dangerous in consumers who are also using alcohol and other opioids, benzodiazepines, or sedative prescriptions. While there are cases of acute and chronic toxicity, kratom has a safer profile than other prescription opioids for most adults and may even be safer to use during pregnancy. It's clear that media has pushed fear over science when it comes to kratom. A harm reduction approach to kratom over forced abstinence respects a patient's freedom of choice when it comes to medical treatment, and should be the goal of every clinician.

CHAPTER 8

POTENTIAL MEDICAL APPLICATIONS OF KRATOM

Patients with chronic illness are on many medications, and that's especially true for seniors. It's the drug-drug interactions that both reduce quality of life and well as cause unintended overdose and death. Respiratory depression from mixes of opioid painkillers, benzodiazepines, and sleeping pills is a common way patients die in their sleep. Studies have shown reducing just one medication patients are on can greatly reduce risk of adverse effects, overdose, and death. If kratom can replace one or more medications in the same way cannabis has, the potential to improve quality of life and even save lives is immense.

Kratom, like cannabis, also has the ability to reduce racial disparities and social inequality in healthcare in the United States. The United States is one of the only developed countries without universal healthcare. Many patients cannot afford to buy their own health insurance, or are underinsured with prohibitively high deductibles for care. Patients cannot afford to go to the doctors, and when they can, they often cannot afford the costly prescriptions prescribed. As an affordable herbal remedy, kratom can provide relief when patients have no other option.

While CBD and cannabis have gained popularity as a way to potentially treat and even prevent some medical conditions due to new research published and extensive media coverage, few physicians and patients are aware of kratom's benefits. The incorporation of kratom into healthcare can yield immense benefits for both patients and society. This chapter summarizes what is currently known about the medical benefits of opioids for certain medical conditions as well as the potential benefits of using kratom if known, and what future research can tell us.

It's important to remember that because kratom is not mainstream medicine, and almost no research has looked at dosing and efficacy for specific condition, that this section will not provide specific dosing or strain suggestions. If you're looking for guidance, the Resources section of this book provides links to the kratom online community as well as consultations with a kratom clinician.

ALCOHOL ABUSE

Heavy drinking is defined as five or more alcohol drinks per day for men and four or more drinks per for women. Alcohol abuse has become a rising problem in the United States due to lockdowns, job loss, and other stressors during the COVID-19 pandemic.[1] It's important that we acknowledge worsening mental health and focus on both alcoholism prevention and alcoholism treatment.

The Pain News Network surveyed of 6,150 kratom users and found only 2.6% were using kratom for the primary purpose of treating alcoholism.[2] It's clear many kratom users decrease their alcohol use, even if they don't identify as alcohol abusers.

ALZHEIMER'S DISEASE

Alzheimer's disease is a form of dementia that primarily impact seniors and is the sixth leading cause of death in the United States.[3] The main cause of this disease is a deficiency in acetylcholine, a neurotransmitter that modulates memory, decision-making and wakefulness. It is also characterized by clumps of beta-amyloid that cause brain inflammation and block signaling between neurons. Finally, neurofibrillary tangles form when tau protein collapses and cannot transport nutrients throughout the neuron, causing cell death.

Patients with Alzheimer's disease show stereotypical symptoms like forgetting things, getting lost in familiar places, or asking the same questions repeatedly. What is less talked about is the mood swings, depression, agitation, and even violence that can even occur towards caretakers as patients don't remember who they are. Alzheimer's patients are usually given prescriptions that balance the acetylcholine system, help with sleep, and reduce anxiety.

Kratom as a neuroprotective agent
Kratom has the power to replace all medications used in Alzheimer's disease, providing a potentially safer solution for a disease plagued by drug-drug interactions and unintended death. Kratom is already used to treat sleep issues, anxiety, depression, and even improve focus. The chemicals in kratom have potent antioxidant and anti-inflammatory properties which can help reduce neurodegeneration and potentially slow down the progression of Alzheimer's disease.

New research further supports the idea of kratom alkaloids as neuroprotective. Minor kratom alkaloid mitraphylline binds to beta-amyloid protein, preventing it from damaging the brain.[4] Mitraphylline and isorhynchophylline, another minor kratom alkaloid, also reduce oxidative stress and promotes mitochondria health in models of Alzheimer's disease.[5,6]

Kratom boosts acetylcholine in the brain

Kratom has immense potential to prevent and treat Alzheimer's disease because of its ability to boost acetylcholine in the brain. The major class of drugs prescribed to treat Alzheimer's disease are acetylcholinesterase (AChE) inhibitors, which block the enzyme that breaks down acetylcholine. These drugs increase the amount of acetylcholine in the brain, restoring brain chemistry and cognitive function to Alzheimer's patients.

Researchers have identified alkaloids in herbal medicines as a potential new source of AChE inhibitors.[7] What's really exciting is that recent research suggests two alkaloids in kratom, mitragynine and mitragynine oxidole B, work as AChE inhibitors in the brain.[8] There is bound to be pharmaceutical interest in developing mitragynine as a prescription drug for Alzheimer's disease.

ANXIETY

Over 19% of Americans had a diagnosed anxiety disorder in the past year, and many more experience anxiety symptoms that are either untreated or don't meet clinical criteria for a diagnosis.[9] Patients with anxiety are often prescribed benzodiazepines like Xanax to handle symptoms, but many also self-medicate with alcohol, opioids, and other drugs.

In patients with anxiety, an imbalance in endorphins in a brain region called the amygdala that handles fear processing may be to blame.[10] When kratom alkaloids bind to certain opioid receptors, it may be able to restore the imbalance in a way benzodiazepines and antidepressants cannot.

Opioids are involved in emotional processing and

strengthen what are called "approach-oriented"emotions (pleasure, bonding, prosociality, and anger).[11] They also weak "withdrawal-oriented" emotions such as fear and sadness. It's likely that kratom, as a mild opioid, elicits these mood-boosting effects.

The Pain News Network surveyed of 6,150 kratom users and found only 14% were using kratom for the primary purpose of treating anxiety.[12] We know that the majority of kratom users use it for pain, but most pain patients also deal with anxiety, making it likely that anxiety would be a secondary purpose for using kratom.

ARTHRITIS

Arthritis is a painful condition characterized by inflammation and swelling of the joints. About 23% of Americans have arthritis, and women are more likely to get the condition than men.

The Pain News Network surveyed of 6,150 kratom users and found that 7.8% of consumers who used it for pain had arthritis.[13] This is not surprising, as kratom contains many anti-inflammatory alkaloids and has been used in indigenous medicine for arthritis. Kratom teas and capsules from red vein strains may be more effective for severe arthritis pain relief than other classes of strains.

Oxycodone, morphine, and hydromorphone are prescription opioids that are sometimes compounded into topical pain relief creams for patients with severe arthritis.[14] Pain relief lotions containing kratom could be a powerful way to relieve joint pain without consuming oral opioids, including kratom.

ASTHMA

About 8% of Americans have asthma, an inflammatory condition where swelling of the airways causes breathing issues, sometimes severe enough to cause hospitalization and death.[15] While it is sometimes seen as a minor problem, asthma actually costs the United States economy over $80 billion dollars a year in medical costs and loss of school and work days.[16]

Mitraphylline, a minor alkaloid in kratom, was found to reduce inflammation in a mouse model of asthma, suggesting it could be a promising therapeutic.[17] In indigenous medicine, Cat's Claw, which is much more abundant in mitraphylline, is used for inflammatory conditions including asthma.

It's unclear how clinically effective taking kratom capsules or drinking kratom tea regularly will be for an asthma patient. Since mitraphylline is a minor alkaloid in kratom, it may take a pharmaceutical extract of mitraphylline in pill or inhaler form to see effects, but this could be a novel treatment of asthma.

ATTENTION DEFICIT HYPERACTIVITY DISORDER

Attention Deficit Hyperactive Disorder (ADHD) is a neurodevelopment disorder that's often first diagnosed in childhood, but it also present in adulthood. The disorder which impact about 3% of adults is marked by poor focus, inattention, impulsivity, poor organization, risk taking and fidgeting.[18] While many patients are put on stimulants like Adderall or Ritalin to improve focus, these prescriptions have dangerous side effects like addiction, weight loss, and insomnia.

Kratom offers a natural way to boost focus and relax, which can help adults with ADHD push through the workday without distractions. Some strains, especially white vein strains, may be too energizing for some ADHD patients and further promote hyperactivity. It's important to experiment with green vein and red vein kratom strains so that you can find a strain that increases focus without making you feel wired. Some patients with ADHD find moderate doses of kratom reduce any overstimulating effects.

AUTISM SPECTRUM DISORDER

Autism spectrum disorder (ASD) is a developmental disorder that includes issues with social, emotional, and communication skills. It impacts over 1 in 50 children born in the United States, and has rapidly increased in incidence over the years.[19]

There is no evidence to suggest opioids, including the alkaloids in kratom, are helpful for patients with autism. In fact, there is an opioid-excess theory of autism, and both pediatric patients and adult patients with autism find removing food-derived opioid such as gluten and casein to be helpful for reducing symptoms of the disease.[20] I discourage use of kratom in adult patients with autism, as it will likely make some behavioral symptoms worse.

There is evidence that opioid use just before becoming pregnant or during early pregnancy may increase risk of the child developing autism by 2.5 times.[21] While I normally discourage pregnant women from using kratom, I also urge women who are trying to become pregnant or not using protection to abstain from kratom use.

CANCER

Cancer is characterized by abnormal cells that growth uncontrollably and spread to other tissues, where they kill surrounding healthy tissue. Cancer is the second-leading cause of death in the United States, and almost 50% of Americans will receive a cancer diagnosis at some point in their life.

Cancer Treatment

Mitraphylline, a minor alkaloid in kratom, has been shown to inhibit growth of multiple types of cancer cells, including human neuroblastoma, glioma, bladder cancer, breast cancer, and Ewing's sarcoma, a rare type of bone cancer.[22,23,24] It was first identified from Cat's Claw, an herb used in Peruvian medicine to fight tumors.

Cancer Pain

Kratom is a potent pain reliever and has been used safely by cancer patients. A recent study in rats even suggests mitragynine, the main alkaloid in kratom, can reduce neuropathic pain caused by cancer chemotherapy through its actions on adrenergic receptors rather than opioid receptors.[25]

Red vein strains of kratom are more potent pain relievers for cancer patients, and the benefits of higher doses for pain have to be balanced with increased risk of side effects. It is important to note there is little research on possible kratom and cancer drug interactions, so be vigilant about potential adverse effects.

Cancer Patients Precautions

Cancer patients struggle with appetite suppression, nausea, and vomiting. Kratom can increase nausea and reduce appetite at higher doses, so it's important to use low to moderate doses for cancer pain and anti-cancer benefits.

Cancer Survivorship

There are over 15.5 million Americans living with a history of cancer. Cancer survivorship focuses on the health and quality of life of a cancer patient after treatment through the end of life. Cancer is a chronic illness, and cancer survivorship is more than just physical health; it's psychological health, social health, and financial health, as cancer causes major changes to a person's lifestyle.

Cancer survivors have to manage their risk of cancer recurrence as well as deal with side effects or lasting damage from their cancer treatments. For example, most people don't realize cancer survivors struggle with fatigue, chronic pain, skin issues, sleep issues, cognitive issues similar to chemo fog, sexual dysfunction, and organ problems. Cancer survivors become socially withdrawn and are less likely to pursue healthy habits like proper diet, exercise, and quitting smoking or drinking. Cancer survivorship programs are often not supported by health insurance, or patients don't know they exist when they are free or reduced in price. Few cancer survivors are supported in their post-treatment phase.

Kratom can help improve mood, fatigue, insomnia, and pain, all health issues cancer survivors struggle with. Endorphin deficiency is associated with cancer growth. With its anticancer effects, regular kratom use could be a tool to prevent cancer recurrence.

CHRONIC PAIN AND NEUROPATHY

Over 20% of Americans deal with chronic pain daily, which limits their function at work and with family. Many chronic pain patients are prescribed opioids, which are addictive and come with the risk of overdose and death. Because of the opioid epidemic, more and more doctors are either refusing to prescribe opioids for more than a week, and reducing or eliminating prescriptions for patients that had been using opioids for years.

For chronic pain patients, there are few affordable and

effective alternatives to prescription opioids. While cannabis products work for some patients, they are ineffective for others, unsafe for people with some medical conditionals, or illegal in some states. Kratom can be a great option for pain patients in states and countries where it has not been banned.

Kratom can be ingested as kratom capsules, kratom powder, or kratom tinctures for pain. It could also be applied topical as kratom lotion to reduce nerve pain. Kratom's number one use is to treat chronic pain. The Pain News Network surveyed of 6,150 kratom users and found 51% were using kratom for the primary purpose of treating acute or chronic pain.[26]

Acute Injury

The Pain News Network surveyed of 6,150 kratom users and found that 11.5% of consumers who used it for pain were using it for acute pain from an injury such as pulling their back out.[27] It's unclear whether patients who consume kratom for acute pain continue to use after their pain ceases, which is one of the issues that is seen driving opioid dependence in prescription opioid users.

Back pain

Over 80% of Americans will experience an episode of severe lower back pain in their lifetime. Causes of back pain include injuries such as falls, car accidents, or strains from heavy lifting, arthritis, fibromyalgia, endometriosis, osteoporosis, scoliosis, and bulging or ruptured disks in your spine.

Unfortunately, back pain is a $100 billion dollar a year industry in the United States, fueled by unnecessary or dangerous surgeries, injections, opioid painkillers, and alternative therapies such as chiropractic adjustments. Many times, the treatments do not help, and in the case of surgeries and opioids, can actually increase pain.

Kratom users overwhelming use kratom for back pain including scoliosis, sciatica and degenerative disc. The Pain News Network reports 38.5% of kratom users use it for back pain.[28] Kratom reduces pain and inflammation, relaxes tense muscles, increases energy, and boosts mood, helping relieve most symptoms a chronic back pain patient deals with.

Neuropathy

Peripheral neuropathy is the most common peripheral (non-brain) nervous system condition, but it is often under-diagnosed and under-treated. Diabetic neuropathy is the most common form of neuropathy, with neuropathic pain seen in about 50% of diabetes patients.[29]

The Pain News Network surveyed of 6,150 kratom users and found that 2.7% of consumers who used it for pain had neuropathy, while 0.4% consumers who used it for pain had trigeminal neuralgia.[30]

DEPRESSION

Depression is the largest global disability worldwide according to the World Health Organization, and over 300 million people live with the condition.[31] Endorphins are released during periods of pain and stress, as well as during rewarding activities like eating or sex. People that are under chronic stress may feel less motivated to pursue rewarding activities, and thus release less endorphins. We know that exercise, which releases natural endorphins, is beneficial for people with depression.[32]

Kratom has immense potential as an antidepressant.[33] The Pain News Network surveyed of 6,150 kratom users and found only 8.8% were using kratom for the primary purpose of treating depression.[34]

EPILEPSY

1.2% of Americans have epilepsy, a neurological disorder characterized by mild to severe seizures.[35] There are many different types of epilepsies, with different causes including mutations in calcium channels that regulate voltage in brain cells.

Opioids may lower the threshold for seizures in patients with epilepsy. The Epilepsy Foundation reports fentanyl, meperidine, pentazocine, and propoxyphene as prescriptions that can increases seizure risk.[36] In healthy patients, high doses of opioids can cause seizures. This is sometimes seen with patients who use doses of kratom over 15 grams, especially in for new users or those who have past substance abuse history.

FIBROMYALGIA

Fibromyalgia is characterized by widespread musculoskeletal pain accompanied by fatigue, sleep, memory, and mood issues. It is often diagnosed by pressing on tender points throughout the body that result in pain upon light touching. Fibromyalgia flares occur when symptoms rapidly increase in severity or number. "Fibro" flares may last for days or weeks and are often dependent on stress levels or triggers like poor diet.

Approximately 10 million patients in the United States have fibromyalgia, and 75-90% are women. While the cause of fibromyalgia is unknown, infections, physical or emotional trauma, and genetics appear to play a role in onset. The Pain News Network surveyed of 6,150 kratom users and found that 9.4% of consumers who used it for pain had fibromyalgia.[37]

One of the main reasons why a patient with fibromyalgia would use kratom is because unlike other painkillers, including opioids and THC-containing cannabis, kratom does not induce sleep at moderate doses. In fact, kratom provides energizing pain relief, helping fibromyalgia patients deal with the fatigue that is often the one symptom their other medications do not help.

HYPERTENSION

Almost half of all American adults have hypertension, also know as high blood pressure. While hypertension is common and often untreated or undertreated, it can damage the heart, leading to heart disease, stroke, and death. Minor alkaloids in kratom including mitraphylline, rhynchopylline, isorhynchopylline, and ajmalicine are suggested to have blood pressure lowering effects. Using kratom regularly may be beneficial for patients with hypertension, especially as a substitute for caffeinated drinks that raise blood pressure.

IMMUNE SYSTEM SUPPORT

Kratom may have the ability to directly treat symptoms of infectious diseases. Kratom has alkaloids that are antibacterial, antiviral, and anti-fungal, fighting potential pathogens directly, while other alkaloids relieving pain and inflammation. Several minor kratom alkaloids have immunostimulant, or immune boosting properties, including isorhynchopylline and isomitraphylline.

COVID-19

COVID-19, short for coronavirus disease 2019, is the respiratory illness that is caused by the SARS-CoV-2 virus. Symptoms range from nothing to fever, loss of sense of smell, severe breathing issues, and even sudden death. Over 500,000 people have died from COVID-19 as of February 2021 in the United States, and 2.5 million worldwide.

Researchers have looked to repurposed prescription drugs and libraries of nutraceutical compounds to find potential immunostimulants, and in some cases, immunosuppressants, to fight the sudden deadly deterioration of COVID-19 patients. CBD and cannabis has emerged as potential therapeutics, but the same research has not occurred with kratom.

Kratom contains many immune boosting and anti-inflammatory compounds, making it a nutraceutical that may have therapeutic value for coronavirus. Kratom alkaloid mitraphylline, which is also in the herb Cat's Claw, shows activity against cytokine-induced inflammation and may be helpful in reducing the cytokine storm that is common in severe COVID-19 infections.[38] Finally, a case study was published where kratom was used successfully for COVID-19 related fever, pain, and fatigue in a patient when NSAIDs were not recommended.[39]

HIV/AIDS

HIV (human immunodeficiency virus) is a virus that if left untreated can lead to AIDS (acquired immunodeficiency syndrome), a potentially deadly incurable disease. There are over 38 million people living with HIV/AIDS worldwide.[40] 1 out of 10 new HIV infections in the United States is in people who inject drugs including heroin, suggesting that reducing needle use will reduce the spread of HIV.[41]

Many kratom users are former heroin users, suggesting that educating heroin and other opioid users abut proper use of kratom in recovery could be a public health approach to HIV. It is unclear whether kratom alkaloids have any antiviral or other health benefits for patients who already have HIV.

MIGRAINE HEADACHE

More than 38 million Americans suffer from migraine headache, a severe form of headache that can several days. Many patients use prescription opioids occasionally to deal with the severe pain. Because of the high potential for addiction and overdose, many patients are looking for natural treatments that are safer but more effective than NSAIDs for migraine pain relief.

The Pain News Network surveyed of 6,150 kratom users and found that 6.2% of consumers who used it for pain from migraine headaches.[42] Kratom can reduce pain, relieve stress, and increase energy, all which are helpful for a chronic pain patient struggling with migraines. But be careful.

Medication overuse headache (MOH) is often seen with patients who use opioids like morphine or oxycodone to treat migraines more than 10 times a month actually making their migraines worse over time.[43] Because kratom contains opioid-like alkaloids, it's important to use lower doses of kratom and to not use it daily, otherwise you may end up trigger migraines with kratom. Do not use kratom while using other opioids, sedatives, or alcohol.

MULTIPLE SCLEROSIS

Multiple sclerosis (MS) is a progressive nervous system disorder that is caused by the immune system attacking the brain, spinal cord, and optic nerve in the eye. Over 1 million Americans are living with MS. Symptoms of MS include weakness in limbs, electrical shock pain, nerve tingling, vision issues, fatigue, slurred speech, dizziness, and sexual, bowel, and bladder function loss.

Kratom contains numerous alkaloids, flavonoids, and other chemicals with antioxidant, anti-inflammatory, pain relieving, and neuroprotective properties. Because MS patients struggle with fatigue, brain fog, and pain, the ability of kratom to relieve pain, boost energy, and improve focus is a combo that can be especially helpful for them.

Patients with multiple sclerosis do not use kratom as much as other patients. The Pain News Network surveyed of 6,150 kratom users and found just 0.6% of consumers who used it for pain had multiple sclerosis.[44] It is more likely that patients with MS do not know about kratom rather than the possibility that kratom is ineffective for them.

POST-TRAUMATIC STRESS DISORDER

Post-traumatic stress disorder (PTSD) is a mood disorder that develops in response to a traumatic event. About 7% of Americans will experience PTSD at some point in their life. The severity or type of traumatic event does not ensure that the exposed patient will get PTSD.

Patients with PTSD are at increased risk of suicide, and more than 22 veterans a day take their own lives. Symptoms of PTSD include mood swings, nightmares, flashbacks to the traumatic event, panic attacks, feelings of hopelessness, irritability, lack of focus, avoidance of triggers, sleep issues, and substance abuse.

Kratom is helpful for relieving symptoms of anxiety and depression at low doses, and inducing sleep at higher doses. Alkaloids in kratom activate alpha-2 adrenergic receptors, which may quiet down a stressed out and overactive nervous system. Alpha-2 receptors drugs including clonidine and guanfacine are traditionally used for reducing agitation and hyperarousal in PTSD patients.[45]

Giving morphine after a traumatic event reduces the risk of PTSD, revealing that opioids can reduce response to acute stressors.[46] While kratom has not been studied in this fashion, using kratom after a traumatizing event may blunt a maladaptive stress response.

SLEEP DISORDERS

Sleep disorders disorders are incredibly common and range in severity from simply frustrating to causing so much chronic sleep deprivation that the patient is suicidal. 30% of Americans have chronic insomnia, which is an inability to fall asleep and stay asleep. 18 million American adults have sleep apnea, which is caused by breathing problems during sleep.

Prescriptions sleep medications like Ambient (zolpidem) are either not effective or cause unwanted side effects, like memory loss after taking it. OTC sleep aids are addictive, and tend to not work after repeated use. Cannabis edibles can help you get to sleep, but you might still feel high when you wake up. So what are your other options?

High levels of endogenous, plant-based, and synthetic opioids can activate mu and kappa opioid receptors to promote sleepiness. It's important to choose the right strain of kratom, similar to using cannabis for sleep. Higher doses of red vein kratom strains are best, as green vein kratom and white vein kratom are more energizing and not right for sleep.

The Pain News Network surveyed of 6,150 kratom users and found only 1.4% were using kratom for the primary purpose of treating insomnia, although it's possible it was a strong secondary reason.[47]

SUBSTANCE ABUSE DISORDERS

About 25% of patients who are prescribed opioids misuse them, and between 8-12% of patients meet the criteria for opioid use disorder.[48] In 2019, 50,000 people died from opioid overdose, which caused doctors to start addressing the opioid epidemic.

Kratom is a safer alternative to prescription opioids and heroin because activation of the mu opioid receptor (**MOR**) does not activate beta-arrestin or cause respiratory depression, overdose, and death by itself. While it would be ideal for patients to first use kratom under a doctor's care instead of addictive prescription opioids, the next best option is for patients addicted to opioids to transition to kratom as a safer substitute. Rodent studies suggest kratom tea does not cause physical dependence, and may aid morphine withdrawal.[49]

The Pain News Network surveyed of 6,150 kratom users and found 9.2% were using kratom for the primary purpose of treating opioid dependence or addiction.[50] It is important to note that kratom users who are in recovery from heroin or prescription opioids often consume kratom at much higher doses than other users, and are at highest risk for drug-drug interactions and adverse side effects.

It is unclear whether kratom is also helpful for addiction to stimulants such as methamphetamine, cocaine, and prescriptions like Adderall. Buprenorphine, a prescription opioid that both activates and block opioid receptors, has recently shown efficacy for both opioid dependence and cocaine addiction. The alkaloids in kratom have not been tested as potential treatments for stimulant abuse, but may be a promising avenue for therapeutics in the future.

TOURETTE SYNDROME

Tourette syndrome (TS) is a neurological disorder usually starting in childhood that is characterized by repetitive, involuntary movements and verbalizations that are called tics. With only 0.6% of Americans having this relatively rare disorder, patients are often stigmatized for saying inappropriate words that they have no control over.

There has been evidence of opioid system dysregulation in Tourette syndrome, including a genetic variation of the *OPRK1* gene that encodes the kappa opioid receptor (KOR).[51,52] Patients with TS that are heroin abusers show reduced tics, suggesting that opioid use may be beneficial for symptoms of the disease.[53] While kratom has not been studied in TS patients, it is possible that the alkaloids in it bay be beneficial.

TRAUMATIC BRAIN INJURY

About 69 million people worldwide experience traumatic brain injury (TBI) each year, which is a disruption in brain function due to bumps or injuries to the head.[54]

Patients with traumatic brain injury (TBI) are at risk for abusing prescription opioids, as more than 70% of TBI patients are prescribed them during their recovery process.[55] Taking kratom for post-TBI pain and well as to to reduce agitation instead of prescription opioids may be a form of harm reduction to reduce opioid misuse.

WOMEN'S HEALTH

There has been little scientific research studies on the effects of kratom on specific medical conditions in women, but anecdotal evidence for the health benefits of kratom on women's health are huge. One thing to note is several surveys of kratom users have found women to benefit from kratom.

A recent study published in the journal of *Drug and Alcohol Dependence* surveyed 2,700 kratom users, 60% being women, and found that they primarily consumed kratom for pain, anxiety, and depression.[56] A survey of 6,150 kratom users by the Pain News Network found 51% used the plant for pain while 14% used the plant to soothe anxiety.[57]

Both pain and anxiety are mediated by the opioid system. Preclinical research studies, which are research studies done on mice, rats, or other animals, suggests imbalances in the opioid system may contribute to many conditions that impact women. What's becoming clearer and clear each day is that because kratom activates the opioid system, it may one day be the target of scientific studies for women's health conditions.

Premenstrual Syndrome (PMS)
Levels of endorphins can drop the week before women's period and for the first days of period flow, a time period often associated with premenstrual syndrome (PMS) symptoms like bloating, pelvic pain, headaches, insomnia, and moodiness. While symptoms of PMS are common and experienced by up to 90% of women at some point in their life, only 3-8% of women have chronic PMS symptoms.[58]

A research study using the Menstrual Distress Questionnaire (MDQ) found that women that did not experience PMS symptoms did not have a drop in endorphins.[59] It's possible that boosting the opioid system may help relieve symptoms of PMS.

Premenstrual Dysphoric Disorder (PMDD)
Women with premenstrual dysphoric disorder (PMDD), a more severe form of PMS that includes severe depression experienced by 2% of women, were found to have lower levels of endorphins throughout their menstrual cycle.[60] It's possible that restoring an endorphin deficiency may improve quality of life for women with PMDD.

Menstrual Cramps and Period Pain
43% of women experience painful periods every month.[61] Millions of women with conditions like endometriosis and polycystic ovary syndrome (PCOS) may experience pelvic pain on weeks outside their menstrual period.

Many women with these conditions take prescription opioids to help manage severe pain, but these medications are dangerous and addictive. Women with occasionally severe painful periods likely don't have access to the same kind of pain management, so what are their options besides taking days off of work?

Endorphins activate opioid receptors to relieve pain and improve mood. Many women find period pain relief from doing cardio exercise and even yoga, which can be traced back to runner's high and the release of endorphins. However, for women with severe pelvic pain, moving out of bed to the gym is not an option.

It's likely that herbal sources of opioids, like kratom, can help women with monthly pelvic pain relief. Kratom is a less dangerous, non-prescription form of opioid pain relief and muscle relaxant for women who have run out of other options.

Labor and Postpartum Pain
In some parts of the United States, 20% of new mothers receive a prescription for opiate pain relievers which can lead to addiction, overdose, and even death.[62] It's known that 1 in 300 women who take opioids for the first time after cesarean birth will become persistent users of opioids, meaning either dependent for long-term or abusing the prescription.[63] It's important that safer natural options for relief be considered, including kratom.

PostPartum Support
Postpartum depression is a period of depression that occurs after birth and is the result of a combination of hormone changes, genetics, sleep deprivation, and stress in 15% of mothers.[64]

Pregnancy, labor, and the postpartum period are full of rapid changes in hormones and neurotransmitter levels. It is well known that endorphins levels are boosted during pregnancy, then peak during childbirth to combat labor pain, and drop postpartum. Because over 10% of women struggle with postpartum depression in the first 3 months after childbirth, it is possible that changes in levels of endorphins may play a role.[65]

A research study by the University of California at Irvine found some women who had elevated levels of endorphins compared to other women while pregnant were more likely to self-report symptoms of postpartum depression when the levels of their endorphins returned to normal.[66] Clearly, more research on endorphins, as well as opioid treatment for postpartum depression, is needed.

While is not recommended that pregnant or breastfeeding women use kratom due to potential for the baby to be exposed to opioids that may alter brain development or body weight, women that are not breastfeeding and struggling after childbirth may benefit from gently boosting their opioid system. Kratom may provide for mood lift, fatigue, and sleep issues that new mothers commonly face.

Menopause
Menopause is the natural end of the menstrual cycle in women, and is defined as 12 months after the last menstrual period. The average age of menopause in American women is 51. By 2020, there will be more than 50 million American women in menopause or post-menopausal and most women are living a third or more of their lifespan after menopause. By 2025 there will be 1.1 billion endocannabinoid deficient women worldwide.

Symptoms of menopause include irregular periods, mood swings, hot flashes during the day, night sweats that prevent sleep, trouble concentrating, vaginal dryness, decreased sex drive, thinning hair, dry skin, weight gain, and loss of bladder control.

Women who are going through menopause and post-menopausal have lower endorphin levels than women who are premenopausal. Even more interesting is that endorphin levels drop even further right before a hot flash, and then rise for 15 minutes afterwards. Could natural opioids provide balance?

Women who have menopausal symptoms are more likely than women who are not in menopause to have chronic pain symptoms and be prescribed long-term prescription opioids.[67] As prescription opioids have the risk of addiction, overdose, and death, safer options for relief should be considered, including kratom.

SUMMARY

Kratom holds immense potential as a natural and safer alternative to prescription opioids and other treatments for a wide variety of health conditions and symptoms. CBD and cannabis were the first big new players in natural remedies. Next came functional and psilocybin mushrooms. Kratom will be the next botanical innovation, and it is wise for patients, clinicians, and retail professionals to understand its full potential before it becomes mainstream.

EPILOGUE: THE SECRET TO SUCCESS WITH KRATOM

I wasn't always good at kratom. In fact, the very first time I took kratom, I broke out in a rash, it was hard to breath, and I was sweating and nauseous. After a couple hours I threw up. After going to sleep, I woke up the next day thanking God I hadn't died.

But as a scientist, I was desperate to figure out what the heck had happened to me. Thoughts ran through my head.

Had I overdosed? I had just taken two capsules someone had sent me. What if they were huge capsules? Nope, I had just taken about 1 g of kratom. A baby dose.

Ok, maybe the kratom was tainted. Maybe the person who had sent it to me wanted me to die (I mean, I didn't know them that well). Omg, Michele, now you're just paranoid! Ok, maybe it was tainted with something like synthetic marijuana and they didn't know? No, that's ridiculous, I trust this person.

Maybe it was heavy metals? I'm seriously sensitive as I was exposed to lead and heavy metals and was hospitalized for it several years ago. I couldn't rule that out.

Was I allergic to kratom? It was a possibility. People who have been smoking cannabis or cigarettes for years can suddenly develop an allergy to those substances. Maybe I'm just so lucky that I'm allergic to kratom my first time using it?

There was only way to find out. I needed to try kratom again. It was 3 months before I had the courage to try kratom again.

I took the same dose, 1 g of kratom, but this time from kratom vendor that was lab-tested so I could rule out being accidentally poisoned by heavy metals or something be laced in it. The capsules were clear instead of brightly colored like the ones I had before that made me sick.

After 15 minutes, I started to feel a bit relaxed, a little happy. After 30 minutes my fibromyalgia pain eased up. No nausea, no racing heart, no feeling like death. Everything seemed ok. I clearly wasn't allergic to kratom.

And then the lightbulb went off. Maybe it wasn't the kratom I was allergic to. Maybe it was the capsules. Capsules can be plant-based, or animal-based and made from gelatin. They can contain fillers or coloring. I have a severe allergic reaction to the food coloring red #40. Even though the capsules had a shell that was half blue, half black, it's possible that some red #40 coloring was used in them.

Long story short, I did some detective work, and in fact, it was the capsules the kratom was capsuled in that I was allergic to. While this was an embarrassing story for someone who's supposed to be a drug scientist and plant medicine expert, I have to also remember that sometimes, I'm just a patient struggling to learn new ways to control my pain and depression.

I'm glad I tried kratom again, because now it's part of my regular pain management protocol and it's made my life so much better. I drink less alcohol, I have more energy and focus, and my fibromyalgia pain is managed more consistently than it was with just THC during the day.

Here are the lessons I want you to learn from my story:

1. Buy from brands you trust. Always check the ingredient label and lab tests before consuming a new kratom product for the first time. If it didn't come with one, don't take it.

2. Use an epiPen, call your doctor, or go to the ER if you think you are truly having an allergic reaction that could be deadly, especially if you haven't consumed enough kratom to warrant the kind of symptoms you are experiencing.

3. Don't give up on kratom if you have a bad first time experience. I know other users that took a bigger dose their first time and felt anxious or too energized. Finding your perfect dose can take some time, and it's best to start slow and build up over time.

4. Not everyone loves cannabis the first (or second or third) time they use it, and the same thing is true with some kratom users. Sometimes it takes practice to be good at plant medicine.

5. Don't like the taste of kratom tea? Try capsules. Allergic to capsules? Try kratom tea or a tincture. There's multiple ways to consume kratom and there's one that will be perfect for you.

6. Get connected with the kratom community online so you can get support if you're confused. There are no stupid questions.

There's no magic bullet to good health or to pain management. It irks me when people say that cannabis or CBD oil can cure everything, or that every single person should use it. There's no one food, supplement, or medication that's right for everyone. And that includes kratom.

Kratom is just a plant, and one of the many tools for wellness. It has the ability to balance your opioid system, fight inflammation, reduce pain, and boost mood. It is still up to you to manage your stress, get good sleep, exercise every once in a while, and eat healthy so your body runs in tip top shape. Otherwise, using kratom while living off of junk food and wine is like putting a bandaid over a bullet wound.

Kratom is medicine, and I'm excited for your journey to healing to begin.

> Good luck,
> Dr. Michele Ross

ACKNOWLEDGMENTS

My life has had many obstacles, but I am as extremely grateful for the lessons contained in each hardship as I am for the once in a million opportunities life has brought me.

To my brother John Osztrogonacz, who died at the age of 20 from alcohol and opioid overdose, all my work is to make sure no one ever has to lose the brightest light in their life to overdose ever again.

To my husband Todd, for saving my life multiple times while I struggled with unbearable chronic pain, and for believing in my dream to launch the first kratom wellness brand for women.

To the producers at CBS and Big Brother, thank you for casting me as the first scientist on reality television, giving me a platform and the power to change people's minds about plant medicine even a decade after first appearing on TV.

To the National Institute on Drug Abuse, Drug Policy Alliance, Colorado Cancer Association, Euflora cannabis dispensaries, and many other organizations and donors who have supported my plant medicine advocacy, education and research efforts throughout the years, none of my work was possible without you.

To the Los Angeles Police Department, who arrested me for being a legal medical marijuana patient in my own home, and the LA courts that made me fight bogus charges for a year and bankrupted me. Thank you for showing me the corruption in government and that every human should have the freedom to consume plants as medicine. Thank you for showing me that we should fight like hell to make sure kratom does not become illegal, and that patients are always protected.

To the American Kratom Association, and all the kratom policy advocates, scientists, brands, and patients that have fought to keep this plant legal and safe for consumption, thank you for keeping me alive. This books stands on your shoulders, as I was too scared to even write it several years ago. Your work convinced federal agencies not to place kratom on the Controlled Substances Schedule, and empowered me to speak up about my experience with kratom. This book is dedicated to all of your hard work you have done, and will continue to do.

APPENDIX: LEGAL RISKS OF KRATOM USE

Cannabis and kratom bear a lot of similarities. One being that one of the most dangerous things about either plant is being caught possessing it or selling it where it is not legal. Before using kratom, make sure it is legal where you live. Most brands will not ship orders to cities or states that have banned kratom. As laws surrounding kratom change frequently, the list below of kratom bans may not be fully inclusive.

STATES WHERE KRATOM IS ILLEGAL

- Alabama
- Arkansas
- Indiana
- Rhode Island
- Vermont
- Wisconsin

APPENDIX: LEGAL RISKS OF KRATOM USE

CITIES WHERE KRATOM IS ILLEGAL

- San Diego County, California
- Oceanside, California
- Franklin City, New Hampshire
- Sarasota County, Florida
- Denver, Colorado
- Parker, Colorado
- Monument, Colorado
- Union County, Mississippi

COUNTRIES WHERE KRATOM IS ILLEGAL

- Australia
- Bulgaria
- Croatia
- Estonia
- Finland
- France
- Israel
- Italy
- Japan
- Latvia
- Lithuania
- Luxembourg
- Malaysia
- Moldova
- Myanmar
- Poland
- Romania
- Russia
- Singapore
- Slovenia
- South Korea

- Sweden
- Switzerland
- Turkey
- Vietnam

COUNTRIES WHERE KRATOM IS LEGAL ONLY WITH A PRESCRIPTION

- Denmark
- New Zealand
- Norway

RISKS OF DRIVING WHILE POSSESSING OR USING KRATOM

It is illegal to use kratom and drive in Alabama, Arkansas, Indiana, Rhode Island, Vermont, and Wisconsin simply because kratom is illegal there. Be careful if you are a kratom user on a road trip and you are pulled over for even a minor traffic infraction. Do not drive with kratom in your front seat or personal belongings, and do not admit to have used kratom or any other substance.

While kratom is legal in most parts of the United States, that doesn't mean you're completely safe. You may still be able to be charged with a driving offense if its use impairs your ability to drive. If you appear to be driving unsafely, you may be subjected to a blood test that looks for evidence of alcohol, illicit drug use, and prescription drug use. Because kratom alkaloids and their metabolites do not show up on these standard 5 panel blood tests, if kratom is the only thing in your system, you will pass your blood test. This means police may charge you with reckless driving instead of DUI, simply because they can't prove you are under the influence of anything.

Keep in mind that if you use occasionally or regularly use

cannabis, as well as kratom, if you are pulled over while on kratom the blood test will say that you failed for cannabis, even if it's been days since the last time you used. This is because THC can stay in your system for 1-2 months or even more after last use. So drive safe as a kratom and cannabis user.

RESOURCES

FOR PATIENTS

Buy AURA Therapeutics Kratom
Dr. Michele Ross founded the first kratom brand for women.
auratherapeutics.com

Kratom Consultation
Learn whether kratom might be right for you with a trained health professional.
kratomismedicine.com/consults

Kratom is Medicine Facebook Group
Connect with other kratom users and get supported.
facebook.com/groups/kratomismedicine

Kratom Research Panel
Contribute to research supporting the medical benefits of kratom. All studies lead by Dr. Michele Ross.
kratomismedicine.com/kratom-research-panel

RESOURCES

Get Weekly Kratom News Updates
Subscribe to the weekly *Kratom is Medicine* newsletter.
kratomismedicine.com/subscribe

FOR PROFESSIONALS

Certified Kratom Coach
Become certified as a kratom coach through the Institute For Plant-Assisted Therapy.
ipatcertified.com/certified-kratom-coach

Society of Kratom Clinicians
Join our nonprofit organization for healthcare professionals using kratom with clients.
kratomclinicians.org

American Kratom Association
The kratom industry trade organization lobbying to fight kratom bans and increase safety regulations.
americankratom.org

IN CASE OF EMERGENCY

Poison Control Hotline
Call 1-800-222-1222 for free help 24/7 in case of non-life-threatening accidental kratom exposure or overdose. Call 911 right away if a person collapses, has a seizure, has trouble breathing, or can't be awakened.

Kratom Addiction Hotline
Call the SAMHSA National Helpline at 1-800-662-4357 for free help 24/7 with kratom addiction or any other substance abuse issues.

NOTES

INTRODUCTION

1. Henningfield, J. E., Grundmann, O., Babin, J. K., Fant, R. V., Wang, D. W., & Cone, E. J. (2019). Risk of death associated with kratom use compared to opioids. *Preventive Medicine, 105851.* doi:10.1016/j.ypmed.2019.105851
2. https://www.wired.com/story/release-the-kratom-inside-drug-culture/
3. Garcia-Romeu A, Cox DJ, Smith KE, Dunn KE, Griffiths RR. Kratom (Mitragyna speciosa): User demographics, use patterns, and implications for the opioid epidemic. Drug Alcohol Depend. 2020 Mar 1;208:107849. doi: 10.1016/j.drugalcdep.2020.107849. Epub 2020 Feb 3. PMID: 32029298; PMCID: PMC7423016.

1. THE KRATOM PLANT

1. Adkins JE, Boyer EW, McCurdy CR. Mitragyna speciosa, a psychoactive tree from Southeast Asia with opioid activity. Curr Top Med Chem. 2011;11(9):1165-75. doi: 10.2174/156802611795371305. PMID: 21050173.
2. Zhang M, Sharma A, León F, et al. Effects of Nutrient Fertility on Growth and Alkaloidal Content in *Mitragyna speciosa* (Kratom). *Front Plant Sci.* 2020;11:597696. Published 2020 Dec 21. doi:10.3389/fpls.2020.597696
3. Charoonratanaa T, Wungsintaweekul J, Pathompak P, Georgiev MI, Choi YH, Verpoorte R. Limitation of mitragynine biosynthesis in Mitragyna speciosa (Roxb.) Korth. through tryptamine availability. Z Naturforsch C J Biosci. 2013 Sep-Oct;68(9-10):394-405. PMID: 24459773.
4. Kerschgens IP, Claveau E, Wanner MJ, Ingemann S, van Maarseveen JH, Hiemstra H. Total syntheses of mitragynine, paynantheine and speciogynine via an enantioselective thiourea-catalysed Pictet-Spengler reaction. Chem Commun (Camb). 2012 Dec 28;48(100):12243-5. doi: 10.1039/c2cc37023a. PMID: 23150886.
5. Flores-Bocanegra L, Raja HA, Graf TN, Augustinović M, Wallace ED, Hematian S, Kellogg JJ, Todd DA, Cech NB, Oberlies NH. The Chemistry of Kratom [*Mitragyna speciosa*]: Updated Characterization Data and Methods to Elucidate Indole and Oxindole Alkaloids. J Nat Prod. 2020 Jul 24;83(7):2165-2177. doi: 10.1021/acs.jnatprod.0c00257. Epub 2020 Jun 29. PMID: 32597657; PMCID: PMC7718854.
6. Ben-Shabat S, Fride E, Sheskin T, Tamiri T, Rhee MH, Vogel Z, Bisogno T, De Petrocellis L, Di Marzo V, Mechoulam R. An entourage effect: inactive endogenous fatty acid glycerol esters enhance 2-arachidonoyl-

glycerol cannabinoid activity. Eur J Pharmacol. 1998 Jul 17;353(1):23-31. doi: 10.1016/s0014-2999(98)00392-6. PMID: 9721036.
7. Russo EB. Taming THC: potential cannabis synergy and phytocannabinoid-terpenoid entourage effects. Br J Pharmacol. 2011;163(7):1344-1364. doi:10.1111/j.1476-5381.2011.01238.x
8. León, Francisco & Gogineni, Vedanjali & Avery, Bonnie & Mccurdy, Christopher & Cutler, Stephen. (2014). Phytochemistry of Mitragyna speciosa. 10.1201/b17666-7.
9. Seo DY, Lee SR, Heo JW, et al. Ursolic acid in health and disease. Korean J Physiol Pharmacol. 2018;22(3):235-248. doi:10.4196/kjpp.2018.22.3.235
10. Liu J. Pharmacology of oleanolic acid and ursolic acid. J Ethnopharmacol. 1995 Dec 1;49(2):57-68. doi: 10.1016/0378-8741(95)90032-2. PMID: 8847885.
11. Mdhluli MC, van der Horst G. The effect of oleanolic acid on sperm motion characteristics and fertility of male Wistar rats. Lab Anim. 2002 Oct;36(4):432-7. doi: 10.1258/002367702320389107. PMID: 12396287.
12. León, Francisco & Gogineni, Vedanjali & Avery, Bonnie & Mccurdy, Christopher & Cutler, Stephen. (2014). Phytochemistry of Mitragyna speciosa. 10.1201/b17666-7.
13. Zeng J, Liu X, Li X, Zheng Y, Liu B, Xiao Y. Daucosterol Inhibits the Proliferation, Migration, and Invasion of Hepatocellular Carcinoma Cells via Wnt/β-Catenin Signaling. Molecules. 2017 Jun 2;22(6):862. doi: 10.3390/molecules22060862. PMID: 28574485; PMCID: PMC6152702.
14. Rajavel T, Banu Priya G, Suryanarayanan V, Singh SK, Pandima Devi K. Daucosterol disturbs redox homeostasis and elicits oxidative-stress mediated apoptosis in A549 cells via targeting thioredoxin reductase by a p53 dependent mechanism. Eur J Pharmacol. 2019 Jul 15;855:112-123. doi: 10.1016/j.ejphar.2019.04.051. Epub 2019 May 3. PMID: 31059712.
15. Gao P, Huang X, Liao T, Li G, Yu X, You Y, Huang Y. Daucosterol induces autophagic-dependent apoptosis in prostate cancer via JNK activation. Biosci Trends. 2019 May 12;13(2):160-167. doi: 10.5582/bst.2018.01293. Epub 2019 Apr 2. PMID: 30944266.
16. Jiang LH, Yuan XL, Yang NY, Ren L, Zhao FM, Luo BX, Bian YY, Xu JY, Lu DX, Zheng YY, Zhang CJ, Diao YM, Xia BM, Chen G. Daucosterol protects neurons against oxygen-glucose deprivation/reperfusion-mediated injury by activating IGF1 signaling pathway. J Steroid Biochem Mol Biol. 2015 Aug;152:45-52. doi: 10.1016/j.jsbmb.2015.04.007. Epub 2015 Apr 9. PMID: 25864625.
17. Jang J, Kim SM, Yee SM, Kim EM, Lee EH, Choi HR, Lee YS, Yang WK, Kim HY, Kim KH, Kang HS, Kim SH. Daucosterol suppresses dextran sulfate sodium (DSS)-induced colitis in mice. Int Immunopharmacol. 2019 Jul;72:124-130. doi: 10.1016/j.intimp.2019.03.062. Epub 2019 Apr 9. PMID: 30978647.
18. León, Francisco & Gogineni, Vedanjali & Avery, Bonnie & Mccurdy, Christopher & Cutler, Stephen. (2014). Phytochemistry of Mitragyna speciosa. 10.1201/b17666-7.
19. Zhang Y, Cichewicz RH, Nair MG. Lipid peroxidation inhibitory compounds from daylily (Hemerocallis fulva) leaves. Life Sci. 2004 Jun

25;75(6):753-63. doi: 10.1016/j.lfs.2004.03.002. Erratum in: Life Sci. 2004 Sep 10;75(17):2143-4. PMID: 15172183.
20. Ito H, Kobayashi E, Li SH, Hatano T, Sugita D, Kubo N, Shimura S, Itoh Y, Tokuda H, Nishino H, Yoshida T. Antitumor activity of compounds isolated from leaves of Eriobotrya japonica. J Agric Food Chem. 2002 Apr 10;50(8):2400-3. doi: 10.1021/jf0110831. PMID: 11929303.
21. de Vries, J.H., et al., *Plasma concentrations and urinary excretion of the antioxidant flavonols quercetin and kaempferol as biomarkers for dietary intake.* Am J Clin Nutr, 1998. **68**(1): p. 60-5.
22. Arai, Y., et al., *Dietary intakes of flavonols, flavones and isoflavones by Japanese women and the inverse correlation between quercetin intake and plasma LDL cholesterol concentration.* J Nutr, 2000. **130**(9): p. 2243-50.
23. Refolo MG, D'Alessandro R, Malerba N, Laczza C, Bifulco M, Messa C, Caruso MG, Notarnicola M, Tutino V. Anti Proliferative and Pro Apoptotic Effects of Flavonoid Quercetin Are Mediated by CB1 Receptor in Human Colon Cancer Cell Lines. J Cell Physiol. 2015 Dec;230(12):2973-80. doi: 10.1002/jcp.25026. PMID: 25893829.
24. Thors, L., M. Belghiti, and C.J. Fowler, *Inhibition of fatty acid amide hydrolase by kaempferol and related naturally occurring flavonoids.* Br J Pharmacol, 2008. **155**(2): p. 244-52.
25. Refolo MG, D'Alessandro R, Malerba N, Laczza C, Bifulco M, Messa C, Caruso MG, Notarnicola M, Tutino V. Anti Proliferative and Pro Apoptotic Effects of Flavonoid Quercetin Are Mediated by CB1 Receptor in Human Colon Cancer Cell Lines. J Cell Physiol. 2015 Dec;230(12):2973-80. doi: 10.1002/jcp.25026. PMID: 25893829.
26. Toker, G., et al., *Flavonoids with antinociceptive and anti-inflammatory activities from the leaves of Tilia argentea (silver linden).* J Ethnopharmacol, 2004. **95**(2-3): p. 393-7.
27. Chen, A.Y. and Y.C. Chen, *A review of the dietary flavonoid, kaempferol on human health and cancer chemoprevention.* Food Chem, 2013. **138**(4): p. 2099-107.
28. Calderon-Montano, J.M., et al., *A review on the dietary flavonoid kaempferol.* Mini Rev Med Chem, 2011. **11**(4): p. 298-344.
29. Wang, C., et al., *Lignans and flavonoids inhibit aromatase enzyme in human preadipocytes.* J Steroid Biochem Mol Biol, 1994. **50**(3-4): p. 205-12.
30. Aiyer, H.S., et al., *Influence of berry polyphenols on receptor signaling and cell-death pathways: implications for breast cancer prevention.* J Agric Food Chem, 2012. **60**(23): p. 5693-708.
31. Nothlings, U., et al., *Flavonols and pancreatic cancer risk: the multiethnic cohort study.* Am J Epidemiol, 2007. **166**(8): p. 924-31.
32. Kim, S.H. and K.C. Choi, *Anti-cancer Effect and Underlying Mechanism(s) of Kaempferol, a Phytoestrogen, on the Regulation of Apoptosis in Diverse Cancer Cell Models.* Toxicol Res, 2013. **29**(4): p. 229-34.
33. Shankar E, Goel A, Gupta K, Gupta S. Plant flavone apigenin: An emerging anticancer agent. *Curr Pharmacol Rep.* 2017;3(6):423-446. doi:10.1007/s40495-017-0113-2
34. Schwarz NA, Blahnik ZJ, Prahadeeswaran S, McKinley-Barnard SK, Holden SL, Waldhelm A. (-)-Epicatechin Supplementation Inhibits Aerobic Adaptations to Cycling Exercise in Humans. Front Nutr. 2018

Dec 21;5:132. doi: 10.3389/fnut.2018.00132. PMID: 30622947; PMCID: PMC6308990.
35. Espíndola KMM, Ferreira RG, Narvaez LEM, et al. Chemical and Pharmacological Aspects of Caffeic Acid and Its Activity in Hepatocarcinoma. Front Oncol. 2019;9:541. Published 2019 Jun 21. doi:10.3389/fonc.2019.00541
36. Tajik N, Tajik M, Mack I, Enck P. The potential effects of chlorogenic acid, the main phenolic components in coffee, on health: a comprehensive review of the literature. Eur J Nutr. 2017 Oct;56(7):2215-2244. doi: 10.1007/s00394-017-1379-1. Epub 2017 Apr 8. PMID: 28391515.
37. Ina H, Yamada K, Matsumoto K, Miyazaki T. Effects of benzyl glucoside and chlorogenic acid from Prunus mume on adrenocorticotropic hormone (ACTH) and catecholamine levels in plasma of experimental menopausal model rats. Biol Pharm Bull. 2004 Jan;27(1):136-7. doi: 10.1248/bpb.27.136. PMID: 14709918.
38. Kiss AK, Piwowarski JP. Ellagitannins, Gallotannins and their Metabolites- The Contribution to the Anti-Inflammatory Effect of Food Products and Medicinal Plants. Curr Med Chem. 2018;25(37):4946-4967. doi: 10.2174/0929867323666160919111559. PMID: 27655073.
39. Kiss AK, Piwowarski JP. Ellagitannins, Gallotannins and their Metabolites- The Contribution to the Anti-Inflammatory Effect of Food Products and Medicinal Plants. Curr Med Chem. 2018;25(37):4946-4967. doi: 10.2174/0929867323666160919111559. PMID: 27655073.

2. THE OPIOID SYSTEM

1. Li, X., Keith, D.E. & Evans, C.J. Mu opioid receptor-like sequences are present throughout vertebrate evolution. *J Mol Evol* **43,** 179–184 (1996). https://doi.org/10.1007/BF02338825
2. Stefano GB, Kream RM. Opioid peptides and opiate alkaloids in immunoregulatory processes. *Arch Med Sci.* 2010;6(3):456-460. doi:10.5114/aoms.2010.14271
3. Brownstein MJ. A brief history of opiates, opioid peptides, and opioid receptors. *Proc Natl Acad Sci U S A.* 1993;90(12):5391-5393. doi:10.1073/pnas.90.12.5391
4. Krishnamurti C, Rao SC. The isolation of morphine by Serturner. *Indian J Anaesth.* 2016;60(11):861-862. doi:10.4103/0019-5049.193696
5. Kapitzke D, Vetter I, Cabot PJ. Endogenous opioid analgesia in peripheral tissues and the clinical implications for pain control. *Ther Clin Risk Manag.* 2005;1(4):279-297.
6. Toubia T, Khalife T. The Endogenous Opioid System: Role and Dysfunction Caused by Opioid Therapy. Clin Obstet Gynecol. 2019 Mar;62(1):3-10. doi: 10.1097/GRF.0000000000000409. PMID: 30398979.
7. Stoeber M, Jullié D, Lobingier BT, Laeremans T, Steyaert J, Schiller PW, Manglik A, von Zastrow M. A Genetically Encoded Biosensor Reveals Location Bias of Opioid Drug Action. Neuron. 2018 Jun 6;98(5):963-

976.e5. doi: 10.1016/j.neuron.2018.04.021. Epub 2018 May 10. PMID: 29754753; PMCID: PMC6481295.
8. Wang D, Tawfik VL, Corder G, Low SA, François A, Basbaum AI, Scherrer G. Functional Divergence of Delta and Mu Opioid Receptor Organization in CNS Pain Circuits. Neuron. 2018 Apr 4;98(1):90-108.e5. doi: 10.1016/j.neuron.2018.03.002. Epub 2018 Mar 22. PMID: 29576387; PMCID: PMC5896237.
9. Dhawan BN, Cesselin F, Raghubir R, Reisine T, Bradley PB, Portoghese PS, Hamon M. International Union of Pharmacology. XII. Classification of opioid receptors. Pharmacol Rev. 1996 Dec;48(4):567-92. PMID: 8981566.
10. Mansour A, Khachaturian H, Lewis ME, Akil H, Watson SJ. (1987) Autoradiographic differentiation of mu, delta, and kappa opioid receptors in the rat forebrain and midbrain. *J. Neurosci.*, **7** (8): 2445-64. [PMID:3039080]
11. Dhawan BN, Cesselin F, Raghubir R, Reisine T, Bradley PB, Portoghese PS, Hamon M. International Union of Pharmacology. XII. Classification of opioid receptors. Pharmacol Rev. 1996 Dec;48(4):567-92. PMID: 8981566.
12. Pradhan AA, Befort K, Nozaki C, Gavériaux-Ruff C, Kieffer BL. The delta opioid receptor: an evolving target for the treatment of brain disorders. *Trends Pharmacol Sci*. 2011;32(10):581-590. doi:10.1016/j.tips.2011.06.008
13. Mansour A, Khachaturian H, Lewis ME, Akil H, Watson SJ. Autoradiographic differentiation of mu, delta, and kappa opioid receptors in the rat forebrain and midbrain. J Neurosci. 1987 Aug;7(8):2445-64. PMID: 3039080; PMCID: PMC6568954.
14. Dhawan BN, Cesselin F, Raghubir R, Reisine T, Bradley PB, Portoghese PS, Hamon M. International Union of Pharmacology. XII. Classification of opioid receptors. Pharmacol Rev. 1996 Dec;48(4):567-92. PMID: 8981566.
15. https://www.caratherapeutics.com/pipeline-technology/kappa-opioid-receptor-agonists/
16. Toll L, Bruchas MR, Calo' G, Cox BM, Zaveri NT. Nociceptin/Orphanin FQ Receptor Structure, Signaling, Ligands, Functions, and Interactions with Opioid Systems. *Pharmacol Rev*. 2016;68(2):419-457. doi:10.1124/pr.114.009209
17. Grösch S, Niederberger E, Lötsch J, Skarke C, Geisslinger G. A rapid screening method for a single nucleotide polymorphism (SNP) in the human MOR gene. *Br J Clin Pharmacol*. 2001;52(6):711-714. doi:10.1046/j.0306-5251.2001.01504.x
18. Crist, R.C.; Doyle, G.A.; Nelson, E.C. et al. A polymorphism in the OPRM1 3'-untranslated region is associated with methadone efficacy in treating opioid dependence. *Pharmacogenomics Journal* doi: 10.1038/tpj.2016.89, 2016.
19. Harris RE, Clauw DJ, Scott DJ, McLean SA, Gracely RH, Zubieta JK. Decreased central mu-opioid receptor availability in fibromyalgia. J Neurosci. 2007 Sep 12;27(37):10000-6. doi:

10.1523/JNEUROSCI.2849-07.2007. PMID: 17855614; PMCID: PMC6672650.
20. Schrepf A, Harper DE, Harte SE, et al. Endogenous opioidergic dysregulation of pain in fibromyalgia: a PET and fMRI study. *Pain.* 2016;157(10):2217-2225. doi:10.1097/j.pain.0000000000000633
21. Kennedy SE, Koeppe RA, Young EA, Zubieta J. Dysregulation of Endogenous Opioid Emotion Regulation Circuitry in Major Depression in Women. *Arch Gen Psychiatry.* 2006;63(11):1199-1208. doi:10.1001/archpsyc.63.11.1199
22. Merenlender Wagner, Avia & Dikshtein, Yahav & Yadid, Gal. (2009). The beta-Endorphin Role in Stress-Related Psychiatric Disorders. Current drug targets. 10. 1096-108.
23. Volpicelli J, Balaraman G, Hahn J, Wallace H, Bux D. The role of uncontrollable trauma in the development of PTSD and alcohol addiction. *Alcohol Res Health.* 1999;23(4):256-262.
24. New AS, Stanley B. An opioid deficit in borderline personality disorder: self-cutting, substance abuse, and social dysfunction. Am J Psychiatry. 2010 Aug;167(8):882-5. doi: 10.1176/appi.ajp.2010.10040634. PMID: 20693463.
25. Prossin AR, Love TM, Koeppe RA, Zubieta JK, Silk KR. Dysregulation of regional endogenous opioid function in borderline personality disorder. Am J Psychiatry. 2010 Aug;167(8):925-33. doi: 10.1176/appi.ajp.2010.09091348. Epub 2010 May 3. PMID: 20439388; PMCID: PMC6863154.
26. https://search.proquest.com/openview/fcb8519dd308690fc095321b28a1b5cc/1?pq-origsite=gscholar&cbl=2032134
27. Collins S, Verma-Gandhu M. The putative role of endogenous and exogenous opiates in inflammatory bowel disease. *Gut.* 2006;55(6):756-757. doi:10.1136/gut.2005.084418
28. Lebovits AH, Smith G, Maignan M, Lefkowitz M. Pain in hospitalized patients with AIDS: analgesic and psychotropic medications. *Clin J Pain.* 1994 Jun; 10(2):156-61.
29. Donahue RN, McLaughlin PJ, Zagon IS. Low-dose naltrexone suppresses ovarian cancer and exhibits enhanced inhibition in combination with cisplatin. Exp Biol Med (Maywood). 2011 Jul;236(7):883-95. doi: 10.1258/ebm.2011.011096. Epub 2011 Jun 17. PMID: 21685240.

3. THE MEDICINAL BENEFITS OF KRATOM ALKALOIDS

1. https://www.asbmb.org/asbmb-today/science/060117/the-science-behind-kratom-s-strange-leaves
2. Andrew C. Kruegel, Madalee M. Gassaway, Abhijeet Kapoor, András Váradi, Susruta Majumdar, Marta Filizola, Jonathan A. Javitch, and Dalibor Sames. Synthetic and Receptor Signaling Explorations of the Mitragyna Alkaloids: Mitragynine as an Atypical Molecular Framework

for Opioid Receptor Modulators. *Journal of the American Chemical Society* 2016 *138* (21), 6754-6764. DOI: 10.1021/jacs.6b00360
3. Obeng S, Wilkerson JL, León F, Reeves ME, Restrepo LF, Gamez-Jimenez LR, Patel A, Pennington AE, Taylor VA, Ho NP, Braun T, Fortner JD, Crowley ML, Williamson MR, Pallares VL, Mottinelli M, Lopera-Londoño C, McCurdy CR, McMahon LR, Hiranita T. Pharmacological Comparison of Mitragynine and 7-Hydroxymitragynine: In Vitro Affinity and Efficacy for Mu-Opioid Receptor and Opioid-Like Behavioral Effects in Rats. J Pharmacol Exp Ther. 2020 Dec 31;JPET-AR-2020-000189. doi: 10.1124/jpet.120.000189. Epub ahead of print. PMID: 33384303.
4. Matsumoto K, Mizowaki M, Takayama H, Sakai S, Aimi N, Watanabe H. Suppressive effect of mitragynine on the 5-methoxy-N,N-dimethyltryptamine-induced head-twitch response in mice. Pharmacol Biochem Behav. 1997 May-Jun;57(1-2):319-23. doi: 10.1016/s0091-3057(96)00314-0. PMID: 9164589.
5. Boyer EW, Babu KM, Adkins JE, McCurdy CR, Halpern JH. Self-treatment of opioid withdrawal using kratom (Mitragynia speciosa korth). Addiction. 2008;103(6):1048-1050. doi:10.1111/j.1360-0443.2008.02209.x
6. Utar Z, Majid MI, Adenan MI, Jamil MF, Lan TM. Mitragynine inhibits the COX2 mRNA expression and prostaglandin E2 production induced by lipopolysaccharide in RAW264.7 macrophage cells. J Ethnopharmacol. 2011;136(1):75-82.
7. Liu, B., Qu, L. & Yan, S. Cyclooxygenase-2 promotes tumor growth and suppresses tumor immunity. *Cancer Cell Int* **15,** 106 (2015). https://doi.org/10.1186/s12935-015-0260-7
8. Andrew C. Kruegel, Madalee M. Gassaway, Abhijeet Kapoor, András Váradi, Susruta Majumdar, Marta Filizola, Jonathan A. Javitch, and Dalibor Sames. Synthetic and Receptor Signaling Explorations of the Mitragyna Alkaloids: Mitragynine as an Atypical Molecular Framework for Opioid Receptor Modulators. *Journal of the American Chemical Society* **2016** *138* (21), 6754-6764. DOI: 10.1021/jacs.6b00360
9. Kruegel AC, Grundmann O. The medicinal chemistry and neuropharmacology of kratom: A preliminary discussion of a promising medicinal plant and analysis of its potential for abuse. Neuropharmacology. 2018;134:108-120. doi:10.1016/j.neuropharm.2017.08.026
10. Takayama H. Chemistry and pharmacology of analgesic indole alkaloids from the rubiaceous plant, Mitragyna speciosa. Chem Pharm Bull (Tokyo). 2004 Aug;52(8):916-28. doi: 10.1248/cpb.52.916. PMID: 15304982.
11. Kruegel AC, Grundmann O. The medicinal chemistry and neuropharmacology of kratom: A preliminary discussion of a promising medicinal plant and analysis of its potential for abuse. Neuropharmacology. 2018;134:108-120. doi:10.1016/j.neuropharm.2017.08.026
12. Obeng S, Wilkerson JL, León F, Reeves ME, Restrepo LF, Gamez-Jimenez LR, Patel A, Pennington AE, Taylor VA, Ho NP, Braun T, Fortner JD, Crowley ML, Williamson MR, Pallares VL, Mottinelli M, Lopera-

Londoño C, McCurdy CR, McMahon LR, Hiranita T. Pharmacological Comparison of Mitragynine and 7-Hydroxymitragynine: In Vitro Affinity and Efficacy for Mu-Opioid Receptor and Opioid-Like Behavioral Effects in Rats. J Pharmacol Exp Ther. 2020 Dec 31;JPET-AR-2020-000189. doi: 10.1124/jpet.120.000189. Epub ahead of print. PMID: 33384303.
13. Kruegel, A. C., & Grundmann, O. (2018). The medicinal chemistry and neuropharmacology of kratom: A preliminary discussion of a promising medicinal plant and analysis of its potential for abuse. Neuropharmacology, 134, 108–120. doi:10.1016/j.neuropharm.2017.08.026
14. Kruegel AC, Grundmann O. The medicinal chemistry and neuropharmacology of kratom: A preliminary discussion of a promising medicinal plant and analysis of its potential for abuse. Neuropharmacology. 2018;134:108-120. doi:10.1016/j.neuropharm.2017.08.026
15. León F, Habib E, Adkins JE, Furr EB, McCurdy CR, Cutler SJ. Phytochemical characterization of the leaves of Mitragyna speciosa grown in U.S.A. Nat Prod Commun. 2009 Jul;4(7):907-10. PMID: 19731590.
16. https://www.nccih.nih.gov/health/cats-claw
17. Dale, Olivia & Ma, Guoyi & Gemelli, C & Husni, A & Mccurdy, Christopher & Avery, BA & Leon, JF & Furr, EB & Manly, SP & Cutler, S. (2012). Effects of Mitragynine and its Derivatives on Human Opioid Receptors (Delta, Kappa, and Mu). Planta Medica. 78. 10.1055/s-0032-1307599.
18. Frackowiak T, Baczek T, Roman K, Zbikowska B, Gleńsk M, Fecka I, Cisowski W. Binding of an oxindole alkaloid from Uncaria tomentosa to amyloid protein (Abeta1-40). Z Naturforsch C J Biosci. 2006 Nov-Dec;61(11-12):821-6. doi: 10.1515/znc-2006-11-1209. PMID: 17294693.
19. García Giménez D, García Prado E, Sáenz Rodríguez T, Fernández Arche A, De la Puerta R. Cytotoxic effect of the pentacyclic oxindole alkaloid mitraphylline isolated from Uncaria tomentosa bark on human Ewing's sarcoma and breast cancer cell lines. Planta Med. 2010 Feb;76(2):133-6. doi: 10.1055/s-0029-1186048. Epub 2009 Sep 1. PMID: 19724995.
20. García Prado E, García Gimenez MD, De la Puerta Vázquez R, Espartero Sánchez JL, Sáenz Rodríguez MT. Antiproliferative effects of mitraphylline, a pentacyclic oxindole alkaloid of Uncaria tomentosa on human glioma and neuroblastoma cell lines. Phytomedicine. 2007 Apr;14(4):280-4. doi: 10.1016/j.phymed.2006.12.023. Epub 2007 Feb 12. PMID: 17296291.
21. Kaiser S, Dietrich F, de Resende PE, Verza SG, Moraes RC, Morrone FB, Batastini AM, Ortega GG. Cat's claw oxindole alkaloid isomerization induced by cell incubation and cytotoxic activity against T24 and RT4 human bladder cancer cell lines. Planta Med. 2013 Oct;79(15):1413-20. doi: 10.1055/s-0033-1350742. Epub 2013 Aug 23. PMID: 23975868.
22. Azevedo BC, Morel LJF, Carmona F, Cunha TM, Contini SHT, Delprete PG, Ramalho FS, Crevelin E, Bertoni BW, França SC, Borges MC, Pereira AMS. Aqueous extracts from Uncaria tomentosa (Willd. ex Schult.) DC. reduce bronchial hyperresponsiveness and inflammation in a

murine model of asthma. J Ethnopharmacol. 2018 May 23;218:76-89. doi: 10.1016/j.jep.2018.02.013. Epub 2018 Feb 10. PMID: 29432856.

4. THE PHARMACOKINETICS OF KRATOM ALKALOIDS

1. Ramachandram, Dinesh Sangarran, Damodaran, Thenmoly, Zainal, Hadzliana, Murugaiyah, Vikneswaran and Ramanathan, Surash. "Pharmacokinetics and pharmacodynamics of mitragynine, the principle alkaloid of Mitragyna speciosa: present knowledge and future directions in perspective of pain" *Journal of Basic and Clinical Physiology and Pharmacology*, vol. 31, no. 1, 2020. https://doi.org/10.1515/jbcpp-2019-0138
2. Maxwell EA, King TI, Kamble SH, Raju KSR, Berthold EC, León F, Avery BA, McMahon LR, McCurdy CR, Sharma A. Pharmacokinetics and Safety of Mitragynine in Beagle Dogs. Planta Med. 2020 Nov;86(17):1278-1285. doi: 10.1055/a-1212-5475. Epub 2020 Jul 21. PMID: 32693425.
3. Kong WM, Chik Z, Mohamed Z, Alshawsh MA. Physicochemical Characterization of Mitragyna speciosa Alkaloid Extract and Mitragynine using In Vitro High Throughput Assays. Comb Chem High Throughput Screen. 2017;20(9):796-803. doi: 10.2174/1386207320666171026121820. PMID: 29076424.
4. Trakulsrichai S, Sathirakul K, Auparakkitanon S, et al. Pharmacokinetics of mitragynine in man. *Drug Des Devel Ther*. 2015;9:2421-2429. Published 2015 Apr 29. doi:10.2147/DDDT.S79658
5. Basiliere S, Kerrigan S. CYP450-Mediated Metabolism of Mitragynine and Investigation of Metabolites in Human Urine. J Anal Toxicol. 2020 May 18;44(4):301-313. doi: 10.1093/jat/bkz108. PMID: 32008041.
6. Kruegel AC, Uprety R, Grinnell SG, et al. 7-Hydroxymitragynine Is an Active Metabolite of Mitragynine and a Key Mediator of Its Analgesic Effects. *ACS Cent Sci*. 2019;5(6):992-1001. doi:10.1021/acscentsci.9b00141
7. Kimheang Ya MS, Janthima Methaneethorn PhD, Quoc Ba Tran PhD, Satariya Trakulsrichai MD, Winai Wananukul MD & Manupat Lohitnavy PhD (2020): Development of a Physiologically Based Pharmacokinetic Model of Mitragynine, Psychoactive Alkaloid in Kratom (MitragynaSpeciosa Korth.), In Rats and Humans, Journal of Psychoactive Drugs, DOI: 10.1080/02791072.2020.1849877
8. Adkins JE, Boyer EW, McCurdy CR. Mitragyna speciosa, a psychoactive tree from Southeast Asia with opioid activity. Curr Top Med Chem. 2011;11(9):1165-75. doi: 10.2174/156802611795371305. PMID: 21050173.
9. Kruegel AC, Uprety R, Grinnell SG, et al. 7-Hydroxymitragynine Is an Active Metabolite of Mitragynine and a Key Mediator of Its Analgesic Effects. *ACS Cent Sci*. 2019;5(6):992-1001. doi:10.1021/acscentsci.9b00141
10. Kamble SH, Berthold EC, King TI, Raju Kanumuri SR, Popa R, Herting JR, León F, Sharma A, McMahon LR, Avery BA, McCurdy CR. Pharmacokinetics of Eleven Kratom Alkaloids Following an Oral Dose of

Either Traditional or Commercial Kratom Products in Rats. J Nat Prod. 2021 Feb 23. doi: 10.1021/acs.jnatprod.0c01163. Epub ahead of print. PMID: 33620222.
11. Kamble SH, León F, King TI, Berthold EC, Lopera-Londoño C, Siva Rama Raju K, Hampson AJ, Sharma A, Avery BA, McMahon LR, McCurdy CR. Metabolism of a Kratom Alkaloid Metabolite in Human Plasma Increases Its Opioid Potency and Efficacy. ACS Pharmacol Transl Sci. 2020 Jul 31;3(6):1063-1068. doi: 10.1021/acsptsci.0c00075. PMID: 33344889; PMCID: PMC7737207.
12. Kamble SH, Berthold EC, King TI, Raju Kanumuri SR, Popa R, Herting JR, León F, Sharma A, McMahon LR, Avery BA, McCurdy CR. Pharmacokinetics of Eleven Kratom Alkaloids Following an Oral Dose of Either Traditional or Commercial Kratom Products in Rats. J Nat Prod. 2021 Feb 23. doi: 10.1021/acs.jnatprod.0c01163. Epub ahead of print. PMID: 33620222.
13. Philipp AA, Wissenbach DK, Weber AA, Zapp J, Zoerntlein SW, Kanogsunthornrat J, Maurer HH. Use of liquid chromatography coupled to low- and high-resolution linear ion trap mass spectrometry for studying the metabolism of paynantheine, an alkaloid of the herbal drug Kratom in rat and human urine. Anal Bioanal Chem. 2010 Apr;396(7):2379-91. doi: 10.1007/s00216-009-3239-1. Epub 2009 Nov 10. PMID: 19902190.
14. Kamble SH, Berthold EC, King TI, Raju Kanumuri SR, Popa R, Herting JR, León F, Sharma A, McMahon LR, Avery BA, McCurdy CR. Pharmacokinetics of Eleven Kratom Alkaloids Following an Oral Dose of Either Traditional or Commercial Kratom Products in Rats. J Nat Prod. 2021 Feb 23. doi: 10.1021/acs.jnatprod.0c01163. Epub ahead of print. PMID: 33620222.
15. Philipp AA, Wissenbach DK, Weber AA, Zapp J, Maurer HH. Phase I and II metabolites of speciogynine, a diastereomer of the main Kratom alkaloid mitragynine, identified in rat and human urine by liquid chromatography coupled to low- and high-resolution linear ion trap mass spectrometry. J Mass Spectrom. 2010 Nov;45(11):1344-57. doi: 10.1002/jms.1848. Epub 2010 Oct 21. PMID: 20967737.
16. Berthold EC, Kamble SH, Raju KS, King TI, Popa R, Sharma A, León F, Avery BA, McMahon LR, McCurdy CR. Preclinical pharmacokinetic study of speciociliatine, a kratom alkaloid, in rats using an UPLC-MS/MS method. J Pharm Biomed Anal. 2021 Feb 5;194:113778. doi: 10.1016/j.jpba.2020.113778. Epub 2020 Nov 21. PMID: 33277117.
17. Basiliere, S., Brower, J., Winecker, R. *et al.* Identification of five mitragyna alkaloids in blood and tissues using liquid chromatography-quadrupole/time-of-flight mass spectrometry. *Forensic Toxicol* **38,** 420–435 (2020). https://doi.org/10.1007/s11419-020-00537-8
18. Kamble SH, Berthold EC, King TI, Raju Kanumuri SR, Popa R, Herting JR, León F, Sharma A, McMahon LR, Avery BA, McCurdy CR. Pharmacokinetics of Eleven Kratom Alkaloids Following an Oral Dose of Either Traditional or Commercial Kratom Products in Rats. J Nat Prod. 2021 Feb 23. doi: 10.1021/acs.jnatprod.0c01163. Epub ahead of print. PMID: 33620222.

19. Philipp AA, Wissenbach DK, Weber AA, Zapp J, Maurer HH. Metabolism studies of the Kratom alkaloid speciociliatine, a diastereomer of the main alkaloid mitragynine, in rat and human urine using liquid chromatography-linear ion trap mass spectrometry. Anal Bioanal Chem. 2011 Mar;399(8):2747-53. doi: 10.1007/s00216-011-4660-9. Epub 2011 Jan 20. PMID: 21249338.

5. THE SAFETY PROFILE OF KRATOM

1. https://www.americankratom.org/vendor/akagmpprogram.html
2. Wang M, Carrell EJ, Ali Z, Avula B, Avonto C, Parcher JF, Khan IA. Comparison of three chromatographic techniques for the detection of mitragynine and other indole and oxindole alkaloids in Mitragyna speciosa (kratom) plants. J Sep Sci. 2014 Jun;37(12):1411-8. doi: 10.1002/jssc.201301389. Epub 2014 Apr 25. PMID: 24659356.
3. Jaishankar M, Tseten T, Anbalagan N, Mathew BB, Beeregowda KN. Toxicity, mechanism and health effects of some heavy metals. *Interdiscip Toxicol.* 2014;7(2):60-72. doi:10.2478/intox-2014-0009
4. https://www.fda.gov/news-events/public-health-focus/laboratory-analysis-kratom-products-heavy-metals
5. https://wonderland-labs.com/how-often-kratom-is-adulterated/
6. Prozialeck WC, Edwards JR, Lamar PC, et al. Evaluation of the Mitragynine Content, Levels of Toxic Metals and the Presence of Microbes in Kratom Products Purchased in the Western Suburbs of Chicago. *Int J Environ Res Public Health.* 2020;17(15):5512. Published 2020 Jul 30. doi:10.3390/ijerph17155512
7. Nacca N, Schult RF, Li L, Spink DC, Ginsberg G, Navarette K, Marraffa J. Kratom Adulterated with Phenylethylamine and Associated Intracerebral Hemorrhage: Linking Toxicologists and Public Health Officials to Identify Dangerous Adulterants. J Med Toxicol. 2020 Jan;16(1):71-74. doi: 10.1007/s13181-019-00741-y. Epub 2019 Nov 11. PMID: 31713176; PMCID: PMC6942072.
8. Lydecker AG, Sharma A, McCurdy CR, Avery BA, Babu KM, Boyer EW. Suspected Adulteration of Commercial Kratom Products with 7-Hydroxymitragynine. J Med Toxicol. 2016 Dec;12(4):341-349. doi: 10.1007/s13181-016-0588-y. Epub 2016 Oct 17. PMID: 27752985; PMCID: PMC5135684.
9. https://www.americankratom.org/mediak/news/akaconsumeralert.html
10. https://www.azleg.gov/ars/36/00795-02.htm
11. https://wonderland-labs.com/how-often-kratom-is-adulterated/
12. Aktar MW, Sengupta D, Chowdhury A. Impact of pesticides use in agriculture: their benefits and hazards. *Interdiscip Toxicol.* 2009;2(1):1-12. doi:10.2478/v10102-009-0001-7
13. Overbeek DL, Abraham J, Munzer BW. Kratom (Mitragynine) Ingestion Requiring Naloxone Reversal. *Clin Pract Cases Emerg Med.* 2019;3(1):24-26. Published 2019 Jan 4. doi:10.5811/cpcem.2018.11.40588

14. Váradi A, Marrone GF, Palmer TC, Narayan A, Szabó MR, Le Rouzic V, Grinnell SG, Subrath JJ, Warner E, Kalra S, Hunkele A, Pagirsky J, Eans SO, Medina JM, Xu J, Pan YX, Borics A, Pasternak GW, McLaughlin JP, Majumdar S. Mitragynine/Corynantheidine Pseudoindoxyls As Opioid Analgesics with Mu Agonism and Delta Antagonism, Which Do Not Recruit β-Arrestin-2. J Med Chem. 2016 Sep 22;59(18):8381-97. doi: 10.1021/acs.jmedchem.6b00748. Epub 2016 Sep 2. PMID: 27556704; PMCID: PMC5344672.
15. Davidson C, Cao D, King T, Weiss ST, Wongvisavakorn S, Ratprasert N, Trakulsrichai S, Srisuma S. A comparative analysis of kratom exposure cases in Thailand and the United States from 2010-2017. Am J Drug Alcohol Abuse. 2020 Nov 24:1-10. doi: 10.1080/00952990.2020.1836185. Epub ahead of print. Erratum in: Am J Drug Alcohol Abuse. 2021 Jan 26;:1. PMID: 33232183.

6. HOW TO USE KRATOM AS MEDICINE

1. Amy Sue Biondich, Jeremy David Joslin, "Coca: The History and Medical Significance of an Ancient Andean Tradition", *Emergency Medicine International*, vol. 2016, Article ID 4048764, 5 pages, 2016. https://doi.org/10.1155/2016/4048764
2. Assanangkornchai, S., Muekthong, A., Sam-angsri, N., & Pattanasattayawong, U. (2007). The Use of Mitragynine speciosa("Krathom"), an Addictive Plant, in Thailand. *Substance Use & Misuse*, 42(14), 2145–2157. doi:10.1080/10826080701205869
3. https://www.cancer.org/healthy/stay-away-from-tobacco/health-risks-of-tobacco/smokeless-tobacco.html
4. Bigliardi PL, Tobin DJ, Gaveriaux-Ruff C, Bigliardi-Qi M. Opioids and the skin--where do we stand? Exp Dermatol. 2009 May;18(5):424-30. doi: 10.1111/j.1600-0625.2009.00844.x. PMID: 19382313.
5. Burkill, I. H., Haniff, M. (1930). Malay village medicine. The Gardens' Bulletin Straits Settlements 6:165–207.
6. Kolesnikov YA, Chereshnev I, Pasternak GW. Analgesic synergy between topical lidocaine and topical opioids. J Pharmacol Exp Ther. 2000 Nov;295(2):546-51. PMID: 11046087.
7. Maneenoon K, Khuniad C, Teanuan Y, et al. Ethnomedicinal plants used by traditional healers in Phatthalung Province, Peninsular Thailand. *J Ethnobiol Ethnomed*. 2015;11:43. Published 2015 May 30. doi:10.1186/s13002-015-0031-5
8. Goh TB, Koh RY, Mordi MN, Mansor SM. Antioxidant value and antiproliferative efficacy of mitragynine and a silane reduced analogue. Asian Pac J Cancer Prev. 2014;15(14):5659-65. PMID: 25081682.
9. Bigliardi PL, Stammer H, Jost G, Rufli T, Büchner S, Bigliardi-Qi M. Treatment of pruritus with topically applied opiate receptor antagonist. J Am Acad Dermatol. 2007 Jun;56(6):979-88. doi: 10.1016/j.jaad.2007.01.007. Epub 2007 Feb 22. PMID: 17320241.

10. Herzog JL, Solomon JA, Draelos Z, Fleischer A Jr, Stough D, Wolf DI, Abramovits W, Werschler W, Green E, Duffy M, Rothaul A, Tansley R. A randomized, double-blind, vehicle-controlled crossover study to determine the anti-pruritic efficacy, safety and local dermal tolerability of a topical formulation (srd174 cream) of the long-acting opiod antagonist nalmefene in subjects with atopic dermatitis. J Drugs Dermatol. 2011 Aug;10(8):853-60. PMID: 21818506.
11. https://www.forbes.com/sites/daviddisalvo/2012/09/22/is-kratom-the-new-bath-salts-or-just-an-organic-pain-reliever-with-euphoric-effects/?sh=7bd9cfcf43dd
12. Vithlani RH, Baranidharan G. Transdermal Opioids for Cancer Pain Management. Rev Pain. 2010;4(2):8-13. doi:10.1177/204946371000400203
13. Ross JR, Quigley C. Transdermal fentanyl: informed prescribing is essential. Eur J Pain. 2003;7(5):481-3. doi: 10.1016/S1090-3801(02)00148-9. PMID: 12935801.
14. Lukasewycz S, Holman M, Kozlowski P, Porter CR, Odom E, Bernards C, Neil N, Corman JM. Does a perioperative belladonna and opium suppository improve postoperative pain following robotic assisted laparoscopic radical prostatectomy? Results of a single institution randomized study. Can J Urol. 2010 Oct;17(5):5377-82. PMID: 20974030.
15. Butler K, Yi J, Wasson M, Klauschie J, Ryan D, Hentz J, Cornella J, Magtibay P, Kho R. Randomized controlled trial of postoperative belladonna and opium rectal suppositories in vaginal surgery. Am J Obstet Gynecol. 2017 May;216(5):491.e1-491.e6. doi: 10.1016/j.ajog.2016.12.032. Epub 2016 Dec 28. PMID: 28040448.
16. Kim HS, Monte AA. Colorado Cannabis Legalization and Its Effect on Emergency Care. Ann Emerg Med. 2016 Jul;68(1):71-5. doi: 10.1016/j.annemergmed.2016.01.004. Epub 2016 Feb 24. PMID: 26921970; PMCID: PMC4939797.
17. Monte AA, Shelton SK, Mills E, Saben J, Hopkinson A, Sonn B, Devivo M, Chang T, Fox J, Brevik C, Williamson K, Abbott D. Acute Illness Associated With Cannabis Use, by Route of Exposure: An Observational Study. Ann Intern Med. 2019 Apr 16;170(8):531-537. doi: 10.7326/M18-2809. Epub 2019 Mar 26. PMID: 30909297; PMCID: PMC6788289.
18. Singh, V., Mulla, N., Wilson, J.L. et al. Intractable nausea and vomiting in naïve ingestion of kratom for analgesia. Int J Emerg Med 13, 42 (2020). https://doi.org/10.1186/s12245-020-00301-0
19. Kathmann M, Flau K, Redmer A, Tränkle C, Schlicker E. Cannabidiol is an allosteric modulator at mu- and delta-opioid receptors. Naunyn Schmiedebergs Arch Pharmacol. 2006 Feb;372(5):354-61. doi: 10.1007/s00210-006-0033-x. Epub 2006 Feb 18. PMID: 16489449.
20. Behnood-Rod A, Chellian R, Wilson R, Hiranita T, Sharma A, Leon F, McCurdy CR, McMahon LR, Bruijnzeel AW. Evaluation of the rewarding effects of mitragynine and 7-hydroxymitragynine in an intracranial self-stimulation procedure in male and female rats. Drug Alcohol Depend. 2020 Oct 1;215:108235. doi: 10.1016/j.drugal-

cdep.2020.108235. Epub 2020 Aug 18. PMID: 32889450; PMCID: PMC7542979.
21. Thériault RK, Manduca JD, Blight CR, Khokhar JY, Akhtar TA, Perreault ML. Acute mitragynine administration suppresses cortical oscillatory power and systems theta coherence in rats. J Psychopharmacol. 2020 Jul;34(7):759-770. doi: 10.1177/0269881120914223. Epub 2020 Apr 4. PMID: 32248751.

7. MEDICAL RISKS OF KRATOM USE

1. https://clinicaltrials.gov/ct2/show/NCT04392011
2. Tanna RS, Tian DD, Cech NB, Oberlies NH, Rettie AE, Thummel KE, Paine MF. Refined Prediction of Pharmacokinetic Kratom-Drug Interactions: Time-Dependent Inhibition Considerations. J Pharmacol Exp Ther. 2021 Jan;376(1):64-73. doi: 10.1124/jpet.120.000270. Epub 2020 Oct 22. PMID: 33093187; PMCID: PMC7745086.
3. Kamble SH, Sharma A, King TI, Berthold EC, León F, Meyer PKL, Kanumuri SRR, McMahon LR, McCurdy CR, Avery BA. Exploration of cytochrome P450 inhibition mediated drug-drug interaction potential of kratom alkaloids. Toxicol Lett. 2020 Feb 1;319:148-154. doi: 10.1016/j.toxlet.2019.11.005. Epub 2019 Nov 7. PMID: 31707106.
4. https://www.painnewsnetwork.org/kratom-survey/
5. Singh, V., Mulla, N., Wilson, J.L. et al. Intractable nausea and vomiting in naïve ingestion of kratom for analgesia. *Int J Emerg Med* **13**, 42 (2020). https://doi.org/10.1186/s12245-020-00301-0
6. Andrew Wong, Monique Mun, "A Case of Kratom Overdose in a Pediatric Patient", *Case Reports in Psychiatry*, vol. 2020, Article ID 8818095, 2 pages, 2020. https://doi.org/10.1155/2020/8818095
7. Ahmad J, Odin JA, Hayashi PH, Fontana RJ, Conjeevaram H, Avula B, Khan IA, Barnhart H, Vuppalanchi R, Navarro VJ; Drug-Induced Liver Injury Network. Liver injury associated with kratom, a popular opioid-like product: Experience from the U.S. drug induced liver injury network and a review of the literature. Drug Alcohol Depend. 2021 Jan 1;218:108426. doi: 10.1016/j.drugalcdep.2020.108426. Epub 2020 Nov 23. PMID: 33257199.
8. Cioe PA, Friedmann PD, Stein MD. Erectile dysfunction in opioid users: lack of association with serum testosterone. *J Addict Dis*. 2010;29(4):455-460. doi:10.1080/10550887.2010.509279
9. LaBryer L, Sharma R, Chaudhari KS, Talsania M, Scofield RH. Kratom, an Emerging Drug of Abuse, Raises Prolactin and Causes Secondary Hypogonadism: Case Report. *J Investig Med High Impact Case Rep*. 2018;6:2324709618765022. Published 2018 Mar 16. doi:10.1177/2324709618765022
10. Tay, Y.L., Amanah, A., Adenan, M.I. et al. Mitragynine, an euphoric compound inhibits hERG1a/1b channel current and upregulates the complexation of hERG1a-Hsp90 in HEK293-hERG1a/1b cells. *Sci Rep* **9**, 19757 (2019). https://doi.org/10.1038/s41598-019-56106-6

11. Lu, J., Wei, H., Wu, J., et al. Evaluation of the cardiotoxicity of mitragynine and its analogues using human induced pluripotent stem cell-derived cardiomyocytes. PLoS One 9(12), e115648 (2014).
12. Leong Abdullah MFI, Tan KL, Narayanan S, Yuvashnee N, Chear NJY, Singh D, Grundmann O, Henningfield JE. Is kratom (*Mitragyna speciosa* Korth.) use associated with ECG abnormalities? Electrocardiogram comparisons between regular kratom users and controls. Clin Toxicol (Phila). 2020 Sep 1:1-9. doi: 10.1080/15563650.2020.1812627. Epub ahead of print. Erratum in: Clin Toxicol (Phila). 2020 Sep 9;:1. PMID: 32870119.
13. https://www.epilepsy.com/learn/professionals/diagnosis-treatment/drugs-their-contribution-seizures/opioids-and-cns
14. Afzal H, Esang M, Rahman S. A Case of Kratom-induced Seizures. Cureus. 2020 Jan 7;12(1):e6588. doi: 10.7759/cureus.6588. PMID: 32051800; PMCID: PMC7001130.
15. Tatum WO, Hasan TF, Coonan EE, Smelick CP. Recurrent seizures from chronic kratom use, an atypical herbal opioid. *Epilepsy Behav Case Rep*. 2018;10:18-20. Published 2018 Apr 17. doi:10.1016/j.ebcr.2018.04.002
16. https://www.marchofdimes.org/complications/neonatal-abstinence-syndrome-(nas)
17. Mackay L, Abrahams R. Novel case of maternal and neonatal kratom dependence and withdrawal. *Can Fam Physician*. 2018;64(2):121-122.
18. Davidson, L. et al. 'Natural Drugs, Not so Natural Effects: Neonatal Abstinence Syndrome Secondary to "kratom"'. 1 Jan. 2019 : 109 – 112.
19. Smid MC, Charles JE, Gordon AJ, Wright TE. Use of Kratom, an Opioid-like Traditional Herb, in Pregnancy. Obstet Gynecol. 2018 Oct;132(4):926-928. doi: 10.1097/AOG.0000000000002871. PMID: 30204686.
20. Yazdy MM, Desai RJ, Brogly SB. Prescription Opioids in Pregnancy and Birth Outcomes: A Review of the Literature. J Pediatr Genet. 2015 Apr 1;4(2):56-70. doi: 10.1055/s-0035-1556740. PMID: 26998394; PMCID: PMC4795985.
21. https://filtermag.org/fears-kratom-pregnancy-overblown/
22. Davis E, Lee T, Weber JT, Bugden S. Cannabis use in pregnancy and breastfeeding: The pharmacist's role. *Can Pharm J (Ott)*. 2020;153(2):95-100. Published 2020 Jan 8. doi:10.1177/1715163519893395
23. https://intermountainhealthcare.org/ckr-ext/Dcmnt?ncid=520732469
24. Matson KL, Johnson PN, Tran V, Horton ER, Sterner-Allison J; Advocacy Committee on behalf of Pediatric Pharmacy Advocacy Group. Opioid Use in Children. *J Pediatr Pharmacol Ther*. 2019;24(1):72-75. doi:10.5863/1551-6776-24.1.72
25. Johnston LD, O'Malley PM, Miech RA *Monitoring the Future National Survey Results on Drug Use, 1975–2016: Overview, Key Findings on Adolescent Drug Use*. Ann Arbor, MI: Institute for Social Research, The University of Michigan; 2017.

8. POTENTIAL MEDICAL APPLICATIONS OF KRATOM

1. Pollard MS, Tucker JS, Green HD. Changes in Adult Alcohol Use and Consequences During the COVID-19 Pandemic in the US. *JAMA Netw Open*. 2020;3(9):e2022942.
2. https://www.painnewsnetwork.org/kratom-survey/
3. https://www.alz.org/alzheimers-dementia/what-is-alzheimers
4. Frackowiak T, Baczek T, Roman K, Zbikowska B, Gleńsk M, Fecka I, Cisowski W. Binding of an oxindole alkaloid from Uncaria tomentosa to amyloid protein (Abeta1-40). Z Naturforsch C J Biosci. 2006 Nov-Dec;61(11-12):821-6. doi: 10.1515/znc-2006-11-1209. PMID: 17294693.
5. Tan MA, An SSA. Neuroprotective potential of the oxindole alkaloids isomitraphylline and mitraphylline in human neuroblastoma SH-SY5Y cells. 3 Biotech. 2020 Dec;10(12):517. doi: 10.1007/s13205-020-02535-4. Epub 2020 Nov 9. PMID: 33194521; PMCID: PMC7652979.
6. Zhou JY, Zhou SW. Isorhynchophylline: A plant alkaloid with therapeutic potential for cardiovascular and central nervous system diseases. Fitoterapia. 2012 Jun;83(4):617-26. doi: 10.1016/j.fitote.2012.02.010. Epub 2012 Mar 2. PMID: 22406453.
7. Konrath EL, Passos Cdos S, Klein LC Jr, Henriques AT. Alkaloids as a source of potential anticholinesterase inhibitors for the treatment of Alzheimer's disease. J Pharm Pharmacol. 2013 Dec;65(12):1701-25. doi: 10.1111/jphp.12090. Epub 2013 Jun 20. PMID: 24236981.
8. Innok W, Hiranrat A, Chana N, Rungrotmongkol T, Kongsune P. In silico and in vitro anti-AChE activity investigations of constituents from Mytragyna speciosa for Alzheimer's disease treatment. J Comput Aided Mol Des. 2021 Jan 13. doi: 10.1007/s10822-020-00372-4. Epub ahead of print. PMID: 33439402.
9. https://www.nimh.nih.gov/health/statistics/any-anxiety-disorder.shtml
10. Winters, B., Gregoriou, G., Kissiwaa, S. *et al*. Endogenous opioids regulate moment-to-moment neuronal communication and excitability. *Nat Commun* **8,** 14611 (2017). https://doi.org/10.1038/ncomms14611
11. Nummenmaa L, Tuominen L. Opioid system and human emotions. Br J Pharmacol. 2018 Jul;175(14):2737-2749. doi: 10.1111/bph.13812. Epub 2017 May 24. PMID: 28394427; PMCID: PMC6016642.
12. https://www.painnewsnetwork.org/kratom-survey/
13. https://www.painnewsnetwork.org/kratom-survey/
14. https://www.arthritis-health.com/treatment/medications/uncommon-prescription-topical-analgesics-arthritis-pain
15. https://www.aafa.org/asthma-facts
16. Nurmagambetov T, Kuwahara R, Garbe P. The Economic Burden of Asthma in the United States, 2008-2013. Ann Am Thorac Soc. 2018 Mar;15(3):348-356. doi: 10.1513/AnnalsATS.201703-259OC. PMID: 29323930.
17. Azevedo BC, Morel LJF, Carmona F, Cunha TM, Contini SHT, Delprete PG, Ramalho FS, Crevelin E, Bertoni BW, França SC, Borges MC,

Pereira AMS. Aqueous extracts from Uncaria tomentosa (Willd. ex Schult.) DC. reduce bronchial hyperresponsiveness and inflammation in a murine model of asthma. J Ethnopharmacol. 2018 May 23;218:76-89. doi: 10.1016/j.jep.2018.02.013. Epub 2018 Feb 10. PMID: 29432856.
18. Kessler RC, Adler L, Barkley R, et al. The prevalence and correlates of adult ADHD in the United States: results from the National Comorbidity Survey Replication. Am J Psychiatry. 2006;163(4):716-723. doi:10.1176/ajp.2006.163.4.716
19. https://www.cdc.gov/ncbddd/autism/data.html
20. Shattock P, Whiteley P. Biochemical aspects in autism spectrum disorders: updating the opioid-excess theory and presenting new opportunities for biomedical intervention. Expert Opin Ther Targets. 2002 Apr;6(2):175-83. doi: 10.1517/14728222.6.2.175. PMID: 12223079.
21. Rubenstein E, Young JC, Croen LA, DiGuiseppi C, Dowling NF, Lee LC, Schieve L, Wiggins LD, Daniels J. Maternal opioid prescription from preconception through pregnancy and the odds of autism spectrum disorder and autism features in children. Journal of Autism and Developmental Disorders. 2018
22. García Prado E, García Gimenez MD, De la Puerta Vázquez R, Espartero Sánchez JL, Sáenz Rodríguez MT. Antiproliferative effects of mitraphylline, a pentacyclic oxindole alkaloid of Uncaria tomentosa on human glioma and neuroblastoma cell lines. Phytomedicine. 2007 Apr;14(4):280-4. doi: 10.1016/j.phymed.2006.12.023. Epub 2007 Feb 12. PMID: 17296291.
23. Kaiser S, Dietrich F, de Resende PE, Verza SG, Moraes RC, Morrone FB, Batastini AM, Ortega GG. Cat's claw oxindole alkaloid isomerization induced by cell incubation and cytotoxic activity against T24 and RT4 human bladder cancer cell lines. Planta Med. 2013 Oct;79(15):1413-20. doi: 10.1055/s-0033-1350742. Epub 2013 Aug 23. PMID: 23975868.
24. García Giménez D, García Prado E, Sáenz Rodriguez T, Fernández Arche A, De la Puerta R. Cytotoxic effect of the pentacyclic oxindole alkaloid mitraphylline isolated from Uncaria tomentosa bark on human Ewing's sarcoma and breast cancer cell lines. Planta Med. 2010 Feb;76(2):133-6. doi: 10.1055/s-0029-1186048. Epub 2009 Sep 1. PMID: 19724995.
25. Foss JD, Nayak SU, Tallarida CS, Farkas DJ, Ward SJ, Rawls SM. Mitragynine, bioactive alkaloid of kratom, reduces chemotherapy-induced neuropathic pain in rats through α-adrenoceptor mechanism. Drug Alcohol Depend. 2020 Apr 1;209:107946. doi: 10.1016/j.drugalcdep.2020.107946. Epub 2020 Feb 27. PMID: 32145665; PMCID: PMC7127966.
26. https://www.painnewsnetwork.org/kratom-survey/
27. https://www.painnewsnetwork.org/kratom-survey/
28. https://www.painnewsnetwork.org/kratom-survey/
29. Dyck PJ, Kratz KM, Karnes JL, Litchy WJ, Klein R, Pach JM, Wilson DM, O'Brien PC, Melton LJ 3rd, Service FJ. The prevalence by staged severity of various types of diabetic neuropathy, retinopathy, and nephropathy in a population-based cohort: the Rochester Diabetic Neuropathy Study. Neurology. 1993 Apr;43(4):817-24. doi:

10.1212/wnl.43.4.817. Erratum in: Neurology 1993 Nov;43(11):2345. PMID: 8469345.
30. https://www.painnewsnetwork.org/kratom-survey/
31. Peciña M, Karp JF, Mathew S, Todtenkopf MS, Ehrich EW, Zubieta JK. Endogenous opioid system dysregulation in depression: implications for new therapeutic approaches. Mol Psychiatry. 2019 Apr;24(4):576-587. doi: 10.1038/s41380-018-0117-2. Epub 2018 Jun 28. PMID: 29955162; PMCID: PMC6310672.
32. Craft LL, Perna FM. The Benefits of Exercise for the Clinically Depressed. *Prim Care Companion J Clin Psychiatry*. 2004;6(3):104-111. doi:10.4088/pcc.v06n0301
33. Johnson LE, Balyan L, Magdalany A, et al. The Potential for Kratom as an Antidepressant and Antipsychotic. *Yale J Biol Med*. 2020;93(2):283-289. Published 2020 Jun 29.
34. https://www.painnewsnetwork.org/kratom-survey/
35. https://www.cdc.gov/epilepsy/data/index.html
36. https://www.epilepsy.com/learn/professionals/resource-library/tables/drugs-may-lower-seizure-threshold
37. https://www.painnewsnetwork.org/kratom-survey/
38. Ferreira AO, Polonini HC, Dijkers ECF. Postulated Adjuvant Therapeutic Strategies for COVID-19. J Pers Med. 2020 Aug 5;10(3):80. doi: 10.3390/jpm10030080. PMID: 32764275; PMCID: PMC7565841.
39. Metastasio A, Prevete E, Singh D, Grundmann O, Prozialeck WC, Veltri C, Bersani G, Corazza O. Can Kratom (*Mitragyna speciosa*) Alleviate COVID-19 Pain? A Case Study. Front Psychiatry. 2020 Nov 19;11:594816. doi: 10.3389/fpsyt.2020.594816. PMID: 33329145; PMCID: PMC7717955.
40. https://www.hiv.gov/hiv-basics/overview/data-and-trends/global-statistics
41. https://www.cdc.gov/nchhstp/budget/infographics/opioids.html
42. https://www.painnewsnetwork.org/kratom-survey/
43. Bigal, M.E., Serrano, D., Buse, D., Scher, A., Stewart, W.F. and Lipton, R.B. (2008), Acute Migraine Medications and Evolution From Episodic to Chronic Migraine: A Longitudinal Population-Based Study. Headache: The Journal of Head and Face Pain, 48: 1157-1168. https://doi.org/10.1111/j.1526-4610.2008.01217.x
44. https://www.painnewsnetwork.org/kratom-survey/
45. Belkin MR, Schwartz TL. Alpha-2 receptor agonists for the treatment of posttraumatic stress disorder. *Drugs Context*. 2015;4:212286. Published 2015 Aug 14. doi:10.7573/dic.212286
46. Szczytkowski-Thomson JL, Lebonville CL, Lysle DT. Morphine prevents the development of stress-enhanced fear learning. Pharmacol Biochem Behav. 2013 Jan;103(3):672-7. doi: 10.1016/j.pbb.2012.10.013. Epub 2012 Nov 13. PMID: 23159544.
47. https://www.painnewsnetwork.org/kratom-survey/
48. https://www.drugabuse.gov/drug-topics/trends-statistics/overdose-death-rates

49. Wilson LL, Harris HM, Eans SO, Brice-Tutt AC, Cirino TJ, Stacy HM, Simons CA, León F, Sharma A, Boyer EW, Avery BA, McLaughlin JP, McCurdy CR. Lyophilized Kratom Tea as a Therapeutic Option for Opioid Dependence. Drug Alcohol Depend. 2020 Nov 1;216:108310. doi: 10.1016/j.drugalcdep.2020.108310. Epub 2020 Sep 22. PMID: 33017752.
50. https://www.painnewsnetwork.org/kratom-survey/
51. Rojas-Corrales MO, Gibert-Rahola J, Mico JA. Role of atypical opiates in OCD. Experimental approach through the study of 5-HT(2A/C) receptor-mediated behavior. Psychopharmacology (Berl). 2007 Feb;190(2):221-31. doi: 10.1007/s00213-006-0619-5. Epub 2006 Nov 11. PMID: 17102981.
52. Depienne C, Ciura S, Trouillard O, Bouteiller D, Leitão E, Nava C, Keren B, Marie Y, Guegan J, Forlani S, Brice A, Anheim M, Agid Y, Krack P, Damier P, Viallet F, Houeto JL, Durif F, Vidailhet M, Worbe Y, Roze E, Kabashi E, Hartmann A. Association of Rare Genetic Variants in Opioid Receptors with Tourette Syndrome. Tremor Other Hyperkinet Mov (N Y). 2019 Nov 22;9. doi: 10.7916/tohm.v0.693. PMID: 31824749; PMCID: PMC6878848.
53. Sarajlija M, Raketic D, Nesic N. Heroin Addiction in Serbian Patients With Tourette Syndrome. J Psychiatr Pract. 2018 Nov;24(6):424-427. doi: 10.1097/PRA.0000000000000341. PMID: 30395551.
54. Dewan MC, Rattani A, Gupta S, Baticulon RE, Hung YC, Punchak M, Agrawal A, Adeleye AO, Shrime MG, Rubiano AM, Rosenfeld JV, Park KB. Estimating the global incidence of traumatic brain injury. J Neurosurg. 2018 Apr 1:1-18. doi: 10.3171/2017.10.JNS17352. Epub ahead of print. PMID: 29701556.
55. Trexler LE, Corrigan JD, Davé S, Hammond FM. Recommendations for Prescribing Opioids for People With Traumatic Brain Injury. Arch Phys Med Rehabil. 2020 Nov;101(11):2033-2040. doi: 10.1016/j.apmr.2020.07.005. Epub 2020 Aug 6. PMID: 32771395.
56. Albert Garcia-Romeu, David J. Cox, Kirsten E. Smith, Kelly E. Dunn, Roland R. Griffiths, Kratom (Mitragyna speciosa): User demographics, use patterns, and implications for the opioid epidemic. Drug and Alcohol Dependence, Volume 208, 2020, 107849.
57. https://www.painnewsnetwork.org/kratom-survey
58. Deuster PA, Adera T, South-Paul J. Biological, social, and behavioral factors associated with premenstrual syndrome. Arch Fam Med. 1999 Mar-Apr;8(2):122-8. doi: 10.1001/archfami.8.2.122. PMID: 10101982.
59. Facchinetti F, Martignoni E, Petraglia F, Sances MG, Nappi G, Genazzani AR. Premenstrual fall of plasma beta-endorphin in patients with premenstrual syndrome. Fertil Steril. 1987 Apr;47(4):570-3. doi: 10.1016/s0015-0282(16)59104-3. PMID: 2952525.
60. Straneva, P. A., Maixner, W., Light, K. C., Pedersen, C. A., Costello, N. L., & Girdler, S. S. (2002). Menstrual cycle, beta-endorphins, and pain sensitivity in premenstrual dysphoric disorder. *Health Psychology*, 21(4), 358–367. https://doi.org/10.1037/0278-6133.21.4.358

61. Grandi G, Ferrari S, Xholli A, Cannoletta M, Palma F, Romani C, Volpe A, Cagnacci A. Prevalence of menstrual pain in young women: what is dysmenorrhea? J Pain Res. 2012;5:169-74. doi: 10.2147/JPR.S30602. Epub 2012 Jun 20. PMID: 22792003; PMCID: PMC3392715.
62. https://www.cuimc.columbia.edu/news/maternal-mortality-may-be-even-higher-we-thought
63. https://www.acog.org/clinical/clinical-guidance/committee-opinion/articles/2018/07/postpartum-pain-management
64. Anokye R, Acheampong E, Budu-Ainooson A, Obeng EI, Akwasi AG. Prevalence of postpartum depression and interventions utilized for its management. Ann Gen Psychiatry. 2018;17:18. Published 2018 May 9. doi:10.1186/s12991-018-0188-0
65. Bloch M, Daly RC, Rubinow DR. Endocrine factors in the etiology of postpartum depression. Compr Psychiatry. 2003 May-Jun;44(3):234-46. doi: 10.1016/S0010-440X(03)00034-8. PMID: 12764712.
66. Yim IS, Glynn LM, Schetter CD, Hobel CJ, Chicz-Demet A, Sandman CA. Prenatal beta-endorphin as an early predictor of postpartum depressive symptoms in euthymic women. J Affect Disord. 2010 Sep;125(1-3):128-33. doi: 10.1016/j.jad.2009.12.009. Epub 2010 Jan 3. PMID: 20051292; PMCID: PMC2891592.
67. Gibson, C.J., Li, Y., Huang, A.J. et al. Menopausal Symptoms and Higher Risk Opioid Prescribing in a National Sample of Women Veterans with Chronic Pain. J GEN INTERN MED 34, 2159–2166 (2019). https://doi.org/10.1007/s11606-019-05242-w

INDEX

7-hydroxymitragynine (7-OH): chemical structure of, 44; medical uses of, 45; metabolism of, 54; potency testing of, 64; production of 15-16; research on, 44-45
alcohol abuse, 32, 109-110, 112, 135, 138
alkaloids: as adulterants, 67- definition of, 14-15; how they work in the body, 39; indole, 16, 49-50; oxindole, 16, 50; production of in the kratom plant, 15-16
Alzheimer's disease, 113-114
anxiety, 32, 114-115
arthritis, 115
asthma, 116
AURA Therapeutics, 6
attention deficit hyperactivity disorder (ADHD), 116-117
autism spectrum disorder, 117
bipolar disorder, 32
borderline personality disorder, 32
buprenorphine, 85

cancer: pain, 118; precautions, 118; survivorship, 118-119; treatment, 32, 117-118
cannabidiol (CBD), 1-2, 5, 14, 38, 83
cannabis (marijuana, THC), 1, 5, 14, 38
chronic pain: acute injury, 120; back pain, 120-121; incidence, 119-120; neuropathic pain, 32, 121
corynantheidine: metabolism of, 56; production of 15-16
corynoxeine: production of, 15-16
Controlled Substance Schedule, 35-36
COVID-19, 123-124
depression, 32, 121
dosing: capsules, 77-78; drug-drug interactions, 100-101; inhalation, 81; leaves, 81-82; powder 79; shots, 80; tablets, 78-79; tea, 79; tinctures, 80
endorphins: deficiency of, 31-32; naturally boost production of, 32-33; production of 26-27

entourage effect, 6, 16-17, 19, 22, 51
epilepsy, 122
fentanyl, 33, 35-36, 71, 85, 108-109, 122
fibromyalgia, 1-2, 4, 32, 122-123
flavonoids, 19-20
heroin, 3, 25, 33, 35, 87, 104-106, 108
HIV/AIDS, 32, 124
hypertension, 123
immune system, 24, 123
inflammatory bowel disease (IBD), 21, 32
kratom: acute toxicity of, 102-103; addiction to: 97-98; adverse side effects of, 88-89; chronic toxicity of, 103-105; driving under the influence of, 109; organic, 69-70; overdose from, 71-72, 102; pronunciation of, 13; recreational use of, 101; storage of, 70-71; tolerance to, 93-96; typical user of, 1; use in children, 108-109; withdrawal from, 96-97
Kratom Consumer Protection Act (KCPA), 61-62, 73
kratom plants: production of alkaloids, 15-16; scientific name, 13-14; strains, 14, 74-77; vein classification, 74-76
lab testing: Certificate of Analysis (COA), 60; for adulterants, 67; for alkaloid potency, 62-65; for heavy metals, 65-66; for microbes, 68-69; for pesticides, 69; for

terpenoid potency, 65; need for, 59-61
lidocaine, 83
methadone, 108
migraine headache, 32, 125
mitragynine: chemical structure of, 15; discovery of, 39-40; medical uses of 41; metabolism of, 52-54, 56; potency testing of, 63-64; production of 15-16; research on 40-41
mitragynine pseudoindoxyl: chemical structure of, 48-49; medical uses of 41; metabolism of, 54; production of, 34,54
mitraphylline: chemical structure of, 46-47; medical uses of 48; production of 15-16; research on, 47
morphine, 36, 108
multiple sclerosis (MS), 125-126
mushrooms, 1, 14
narcotics, 35-36
nausea, 68-69, 87, 89-92, 102, 118
neonatal abstinence syndrome (NAS), 105-106
opioids: definition, 33; dependence on, 4; food-derived, 34-35; history of use, 25; genetics of opioid system, 30-31; opiates, 33-35; overdose from, 3; receptors, 27-29; recovery from, 101-102, system function, 23-26
opium, 26, 33, 35, 44, 87, 91
oxycodone (OxyContin, Percocet), 36, 108

INDEX

paynantheine: chemical structure of, 42; medical uses of 43; metabolism of, 55; production of 15-16; research on 42-43
phenols, 20-21
post-traumatic stress disorder (PTSD), 32, 126
saponins, 18-19
schizophrenia, 32
sleep: apnea, 127; insomnia, 26, 127
speciociliatine: chemical structure of, 45-46; medical uses of, 46; metabolism of, 55-56; production of 15-16; research on, 46
speciogynine: chemical structure of, 43; medical uses of, 44; metabolism of, 55; production of 15-16; research on 43-44
speciophylline: production of 15-16
substance abuse: stimulants, 128; opioids, 3, 32, 127-128
suppositories, 87-88
tannins, 21
temporomandibular joint syndrome (TMJ), 32
terpenoids: definition of, 17-18; potency testing for: 65
tobacco, 81-82
topicals: bath bombs, 84; bath salts, 84-85; pain relief cream, 82-83; skincare 83; soap, 83-84; transdermal patches, 85-87
Tourette syndrome, 128-129
traumatic brain injury (TBI), 129
women's health: breastfeeding, 107-108; endometriosis, 130; kratom use, 129; labor pain, 131; menstrual cramps, 130-131; menopause, 132-133; period pain, 130-131; polycystic ovary syndrome (PCOS), 130; postpartum depression, 131-132; postpartum pain, 131; pregnancy, 105-107; premenstrual disorder (PMS), 130; premenstrual dysphoric disorder (PMDD), 130

ABOUT THE AUTHOR

Dr. Michele Ross, PhD, MBA, is a leading expert in plant medicine and the founder of the first kratom wellness brand for women, AURA Therapeutics. She has trained thousands of healthcare professionals and patients around the world on the medical benefits of CBD, cannabis, kratom, and mushrooms. She has published five books, including *Vitamin Weed*, *CBD Oil For Health*, *Journal Yourself To Health*, and *Train Your Brain To Get Thin*. Dr. Ross received her doctorate in Neuroscience from the University of Texas Southwestern Medical Center at Dallas. She was the first scientist in the world to star on reality television on the hit CBS show *Big Brother 11*. Stay connected at drmicheleross.com.

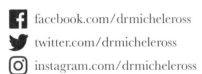

facebook.com/drmicheleross
twitter.com/drmicheleross
instagram.com/drmicheleross

ALSO BY DR. MICHELE ROSS

CBD OIL FOR HEALTH

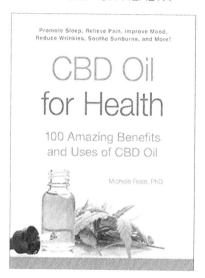

In *CBD Oil for Health* you will find 100 different uses and recipes for CBD oil including health and beauty recipes. Neuroscientist Dr. Ross provides information about CBD oil including as why it's legal, how it works in the body, its health benefits, proper dosage, and more. This detailed resource will allow you to use your CBD oil with confidence.

VITAMIN WEED: A 4-STEP PLANT TO PREVENT AND REVERSE ENDOCANNABINOID DEFICIENCY

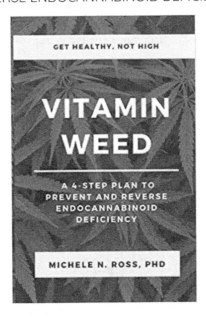

In *Vitamin Weed*, neuroscientist Dr. Michele Ross outlines how restoring balance to your ECS is the key to fighting inflammation, pain, aging, and even cancer. You'll learn how to get rid of aches and pains, boost energy and reduce stress, improve your mood and find motivation for life, reduce dependence on prescription pills and drugs, and teach your body how to heal itself.

JOURNAL YOURSELF TO HEALTH

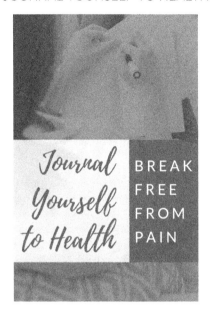

Journal Yourself To Health contains the 30 journal prompts that healed neuroscientist and Big Brother star Dr. Michele Ross. This workbook transformed her life from a full-time patient, living in ERs, to exploring the world as an international speaker. These prompts are designed to elevate your vibration into full alignment with the healthiest version of yourself *today*. As a bonus, 31 healing mantras you can say every day to relieve stress and guide your cells to heal yourself are also included.

TRAIN YOUR BRAIN TO GET THIN

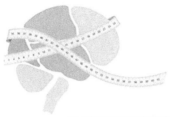

PRIME YOUR GRAY CELLS FOR
WEIGHT LOSS, WELLNESS, AND EXERCISE

TRAIN YOUR BRAIN TO Get Thin

Melinda Boyd, MPH, MHR, RD with Michele Noonan, PhD

Train Your Brain to Get Thin combines the latest research in both neuroscience and human behavior to give you the brain-changing program you need to get fit, look good, and feel great–for life! You'll learn how to control emotional eating, get addicted to exercise and control hunger levels in this book written by neuroscientist Dr. Michele Noonan Ross and Melinda Boyd.

Made in United States
North Haven, CT
01 June 2025